To Cantor Hal Rifkin,
 Our wonderful, gifted chazan. Your
talent as a cantor, and your friendly,
kind-hearted demeanor, are an inspiration
to all of us. Hope you enjoy the stories!
Best wishes to you, to Marti and your
wonderful family. Your friend,
           Paul Brief
          Nov 2012

HOOTCH 8
A Combat Surgeon Remembers Vietnam

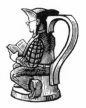

L. Paul Brief, MD

HOOTCH 8

A Combat Surgeon Remembers Vietnam

Hootch 8
A Combat Surgeon Remembers Vietnam

First Edition 2012

The Toby Press LLC
POB 8531, New Milford, CT 06776, USA
& POB 4044, Jerusalem 91040, Israel
www.tobypress.com

ISBN 978 1 59264 365 3, *hardcover*

A CIP catalogue record for this title is
available from the British Library

Printed and bound in the United States

*To the men of Hootch 8 and First Medical Battalion,
without whose friendship, support, and good cheer,
I would surely have come home in a strait jacket.*

Contents

Author's Note

In Vietnam, officer lodgings were typically referred to as "hootches." Sturdy framed wooden structures built on wood posts with plywood floors, screened walls, and corrugated metal roofs, they measured approximately twenty by thirty feet, with front and rear doors that could be accessed by several wooden steps. Home to half a dozen men, most hootches had large underground bunkers eight feet deep adjacent to the rear door. During times of high alert or direct enemy attack, officers would low-crawl out the rear door and slip into the bunker with their weapons. Hootches were arranged in rows on either side of a plank walkway, each hootch wired for electricity and equipped with a "squawkbox" intercom system for rapid notification by the ER staff. Hootches had no plumbing as all communal bathrooms, showers, and toilet facilities were located separately.

Prologue

At the ripe old age of thirty, my medical training ended abruptly when I was thrown headlong into military duty in Vietnam. In a matter of days, I went from being an orthopedic surgery resident in New York City, where the worst thing that could happen to me was getting yelled at by the chief, straight to combat surgery in Danang, where the worst thing that could happen was getting my head blown off by a Vietcong rocket.

By then, the long and arduous minefield of surgical training had consumed nearly a third of my life. I suppose I learned orthopedics well enough, but I also learned that there was no limit to how cruel and tyrannical some surgeons could be. Irreverent, rebellious, and blessed with resentment of authority in any form, I found myself unable to respond to the mistreatment with mere silence, and often made attempts at humor. But as I discovered, reacting to a surgeon-tyrant with levity can have dire consequences. Still, it was preferable to remaining silent, which encouraged even more abuse.

In my first month as a rotating surgical intern at Mt. Sinai Hospital in New York City, I had the privilege of assisting the redoubtable Dr. Sidney Garlock. Pompous and terrifying, he enjoyed peppering his subordinates with rapid-fire questions such as: "Son, why is it my incisions don't bleed?" Having no idea what the answer was, I blurted out: "They're afraid to, sir!"

"Why you impertinent young man, get out! Leave this operating room at once!"

I left, but as he had no idea who I was behind my surgical mask, I ended up operating with him again a couple days later. This time I was careful to refrain from speaking. Later that year I was assisting Dr. Arthur Ship, chief of plastic surgery at The Hospital for Joint Diseases in Harlem, when he asked me to suture shut one of the tissue layers. As I was doing my best to stitch away, Dr. Ship remarked, "Brief, you should really learn to suture a little better."

"Yes sir," I replied, "I believe that's what I'm here for."

"You're absolutely right," he said, laughing. "Here, let me show you how it's done." He went on to demonstrate his flowing, expert suturing technique, which I use to this day.

As the year progressed, I got to work with most of the surgeons at our hospital, and I couldn't help noticing that two of them seemed to despise each other. Although they were both capable and successful doctors, they tended to wander into the OR while the other was operating to make snide or critical remarks. One day as I was assisting Dr. Frank, his arch-enemy Dr. Mintz walked in and noticed that Dr. Frank was using a magnificent new set of gold-plated surgical instruments, which he'd had custom-made.

Standing behind me watching his colleague operate, Dr. Mintz leaned over and whispered in Yiddish loud enough for all to hear: "*Az min hott nischt goldene hendt darf min nitzen goldene kaylim,*" "If you don't have golden hands, might as well use golden instruments." Then he walked out, leaving Dr. Frank fuming and me smiling behind my mask.

Some surgeons were known for abusing their subordinates, whether nurses, technicians or doctors. Dr. Mark Lazansky was a brilliant orthopedic surgeon, and the first to import the technique of total hip replacement (THR) from England to the U.S. While a perfect gentleman outside the OR, Dr. Lazansky did a Dr. Jekyll-Mr. Hyde turnabout when he operated, suddenly insulting and disparaging everyone around him.

Lazansky's behavior in the OR was such that upperclassmen residents assigned to him for three-month rotations would typically quit after four to six weeks, asking to be re-assigned.

When my turn came, I found I enjoyed watching and learning from him. Despite the bullying, I immediately recognized his surgical brilliance. But after a full month of humiliation and sarcasm, my patience had worn thin. Following a particularly difficult morning peppered with insults, I confronted him.

"Dr. Lazansky, I believe I've been a good resident, preparing your patients for surgery then following them diligently until discharge. I am never late and I'm always here to assist you, but I feel that if you continue to treat me the way you do, with insults and no regard for my feelings, I'll be forced to do as my predecessors and ask to be re-assigned. I'm being mistreated and I think I deserve better."

He appeared momentarily shocked, then quickly regained his composure.

"You know Brief, you're right. You do deserve better, and I apologize."

The next morning, after his THR patient had been prepped for surgery, he handed me the knife and said, "Go ahead, you do the case. I'll take you through it step by step." It was the first time I'd ever heard of Lazansky giving a resident such an opportunity. Luckily, I had been watching him carefully for a month and with his guidance, the case came out nicely. Over the next two months he allowed me to perform a majority of his surgeries, which not only enabled me to gain a good deal of confidence in THR, but also paved the way for a friendship.

But to this day, no humiliation inflicted upon me compares to the one I suffered at the hands of the chief of orthopedics in 1969, only a couple of weeks before my graduation and about a month before I left for Vietnam. It was so hurtful that I'd rather not name him and just refer to him as Dr. P.

Dr. McKinley Wiles was a black urologist at our hospital who was known not only for his skill, but for his compassionate bedside manner. Before surgery, Dr. Wiles would stand next to his patient with a Bible and they would pray together, eyes closed, each placing a hand on the book. It was a touching, unforgettable scene that I witnessed many times during my residency. Unfortunately, in 1969, Dr. Wiles fell gravely ill with a malignancy and ended up hospitalized under the care of Dr. P. because of multiple vertebral fractures from metastatic cancer. As a senior resident in the last weeks of training, I was then personal assistant to the chief and made rounds on all his patients twice a day, overseeing their care and reporting to the boss daily.

One morning as we were rounding at the usual 6 A.M. with Dr. P. and his entourage of students, nurses, and residents, we all stopped at the bedside of Dr. Wiles, whose condition by then appeared terminal. The chief asked me to report on the patient's progress and I gave him a clear and concise report, as I had reviewed the chart earlier that morning. Then Dr. P. turned to me and said:

"Brief, what's the serum calcium?"

"It's a bit high, sir, 12.9."

"And when was that done?"

"Two days ago, sir," I replied.

"Two days ago? Did you say two days ago?"

"Yes, sir."

"That's outrageous! You mean to tell me this man hasn't had his serum calcium measured in forty-eight hours? And when is his next calcium due?"

"Tomorrow morning, sir. We measure his calcium every seventy-two hours as per protocol."

"That's infuriating, Brief! And don't give me that crap about protocol! You know very well that a man as sick as Dr. Wiles should have his calcium tested daily!"

"Sir, I checked with Oncology, who advised me that..."

"Stop it, Brief. Stop right there!"

He was obviously furious.

"You are incompetent!" he screamed. "You embarrass this department! And I hope, I sincerely hope, that someday when *you* are lying on your deathbed, some resident takes better care of you than you are taking care of this man!"

With that, he stormed out, his entire entourage following sheepishly behind him, as I stood there, stunned. I broke my back for this man, made rounds on his patients every day at 5 A.M., knew their cases by heart, and now this?

As I stood there at the bedside, I felt a touch on my hand and looked down to see that Dr. Wiles had placed his hand on mine. He motioned for me to come closer and whispered in his kind but weakened voice: "Dr. Brief, I disagree. I think you are taking care of me very well indeed and I thank you for all you do. Please come back this afternoon. I've got something I'd like to give you."

When I came back later that day, Dr. Wiles handed me a package and asked me to open it. It was his Bible, the one he used to pray with his patients before surgery. The inside of the front cover was inscribed: *To my esteemed friend Paul Brief. McKinley Wiles, June 16, 1969.*

I will never forget the kindness extended to me that day by Dr. Wiles, who died the following week surrounded by his family. His Bible remains one of my most precious possessions.

Chapter One

Goodbye, New York

'R un to Canada?" I asked.

"Of course run to Canada, you idiot! What are you doing going to Vietnam? It's a slaughter-fest out there, you'll get your ass shot off! And besides, where am I going to get some decent wine around here if you fly the coop?"

My friend Phil Neuberg was never at a loss for words. A recent graduate of Columbia Law School with a good job, Phil had been fortunate enough to draw a very high number in the draft lottery, virtually ensuring his freedom from military service forever. I was not so lucky. Here I was in April 1969, two months away from the end of my residency training in orthopedic surgery, and suddenly I was a commissioned officer in the United States Navy.

Back in 1964, I had signed up for the Berry Plan, whereby the Navy would allow me to complete my residency training in exchange for two years of active duty immediately afterward. Who thought in 1964 that we would be in this war for another decade? And why had I chosen the Navy? For no reason other than that I loved the dress blue uniform. Did I know that all Marine Corps doctors came from the Navy? I did not. (Marines are strictly combatants. All of their ancillary personnel such as doctors, dentists, nurses, lawyers, clergy, and administrators come from the Navy.) So here I was assigned to Charlie Company, First Medical Battalion Hospital, First Marine Division, in Danang, Republic of Vietnam. Totally screwed, no way I could get out of it. But... run to Canada? As a commissioned naval officer with the rank of lieutenant, escaping to Canada would qualify as a form of desertion.

"Sorry, Phil, but you know I'm a naturalized American citizen since 1961, you know I made a commitment to give the Navy two years, and now I have to go. I can't run. Besides, somebody has to care for those poor injured bastards over there, might as well be me."

"Somebody? Somebody?" he shouted back. "Paul, you *are* crazy! They've got career doctors in the service who love that crap, they don't need you civilian docs over there! You ask me, Toronto looks more beautiful by the minute!"

Phil was a good friend who cared about me, but he was wrong. I could not be a deserter. I also knew that if I ran to Canada or elsewhere to avoid service in Vietnam, I would scuttle my future in the US. I could never practice medicine in this country with a clear conscience, and would feel an awful guilt each time I saw a wounded veteran crutch-walking down the street. I would embarrass my parents, my younger brother and sister. But most of all, running would make me feel ashamed, like a coward.

"Thanks, Phil, but no thanks. Toronto may be a beautiful place, but not for me."

Instead, I suggested we go pick up our dates, pop open a couple of good bottles, and see what happens. I lived in a small but cozy studio apartment on East 88th Street, which Phil wanted to sublet when I left come July. My date Marina lived on 63rd Street and we had arranged for a double date with her roommate Natalie. Marina was smart, blonde, shapely, and very proud of her ample bosom. Each time she leaned forward or crossed her arms, her breasts would bulge temptingly enough to make eyes pop. Blessed with a brilliant smile and an infectious laugh, she was an up-and-coming fashion designer who dressed beautifully. Her roommate Natalie, quiet and dark, took an immediate liking to Phil. Why not? Tall, handsome, funny, and a lawyer, he had an open, carefree way about him which put women at ease.

"Puligny-Montrachet 1965, ladies, one of my favorite white wines," I said, popping open the bottle on Marina's coffee table and pouring some for each of us.

"Would anybody prefer red? I have a nice Chateau Talbot 1963," I offered.

"Just pour, Brief, don't lecture," interrupted Phil. "The man likes to talk about wine even more than he likes to drink it!"

Marina was a gifted athlete with great stamina, and sex with her was bit like white water rafting: exhilarating, noisy, and tiring. A distance runner and aerobic dancer, she often left me breathless. Our activities typically extended through the night, with me dashing off to the hospital before 5 A.M., and her leaving for work later in the morning. Unencumbered by any squeamishness about nudity, she liked to walk around my apartment undressed, especially since I made no effort to conceal my admiration for her near-perfect "Vargas Girl" shape.

But she was not my steady girlfriend for a number of reasons. First, we both knew I was going off to war in a matter of months, making my future uncertain. Second, Marina already had a steady boyfriend who wanted to marry her, a prospect which at the age of twenty-four, she found distasteful. But the real reason, I admit, was the sheer number of options available to a twenty-nine-year-old bachelor in 1969 New York City, smack in the middle of the sexual revolution. The parties, the bars, the parks, even the work places offered up a dizzying array of romantic possibilities I found myself unable to resist. My dating choices seemed to be unlimited, and with most of the women I met being on "the pill," there was little to worry about. Still, I was always discreet. I never boasted or joked about my so-called sexual conquests. I would politely decline to name names or discuss any sexual details when asked, and after a while my good friends stopped asking.

How could I say goodbye to my life in New York? How could I part with my friends, my colleagues, my single life? I was aware that I was leaving for a distant and hostile country with no certainty of a safe return. Should I write a long farewell letter and mail out copies?

In May 1969 I finally decided that I needed to have one last huge party and invite everyone I knew, without exception. I decided to go all out. After all, who knew when I would have such an opportunity again? The party would be held at my apartment, with the best wine and food I could afford. All my pals from college, medical school, orthopedic residency, and bachelorhood would be invited. I faced a dilemma about which women to invite, and in the end, resolved to invite them all: every woman I was currently dating, had previously dated, or hoped to date in the future. One might wonder how I could invite them all. Wouldn't they be sore at me? But when I contacted nearly every woman I had ever gone out with and invited her to my farewell party, the vast majority accepted. Of course, they were well aware my buddies would all be there and, anyway, you never know who you'll meet at a New York City party.

On Saturday night, June 25, 1969, more than one hundred and fifty people in tuxedos and evening gowns wandered in and out of my apartment. Why had I asked my friends to come in black tie? If I were to get my ass shot off in Vietnam and never return, I figured the least my friends could do was look their best to see me off.

It was mayhem, it was pandemonium, it was wonderful. Wall to wall hugs, kisses, few if any tears, with music, food, wine, laughter, and one four-foot bottle of Chianti, which my brother Ben accidentally danced into and broke, releasing an overwhelming aroma of cheap red wine into the place. It was probably the most fun I've ever had in my life. No speeches, no lengthy goodbyes, no gifts. By the wee hours, everybody had gone, while Marina, Phil, and Ben stayed to help me clean up.

I slept for the next two days and was awakened by a loud knock on my door. A Federal Express envelope had arrived containing my orders from the United States Navy Adjutant General: I was to report on July 19, 1969, to the United States Marine Corps base at Camp Pendleton, California for boot camp training.

Chapter Two

'This child saved us all'

In order to understand the sense of duty I felt toward my adopted country, you'd have to know a little bit about my past. I was born in Soroca, Romania on July 11, 1939 to Itta Libman and Sigmund Brief. For some reason, it was my maternal grandfather Bentzion Libman who was tasked with officially registering my birth. As the story goes, it took him a full three days to make his way to City Hall, so that my official date of birth is July 14, 1939.

Soroca, which was also my mother's birthplace, was a small town of some four thousand souls in Bessarabia, a Russian-speaking province of Romania. My father was from Chernowitz in Bucovina, a German-speaking province formerly part of the Hapsburg Empire, some fifty miles away. When World War II broke out on September 1, 1939, just six weeks after my birth, my parents fled westward. My mother would never see her parents again.

During the war, we were wind-tossed all over Romania, running from town to town, from one refugee camp to the next. At some point, my father fell ill with spotted typhus, an epidemic that by the end of the war would claim tens of thousands of lives. Even with a sick husband, my mother managed to drag us from place to place, all the while nurturing and protecting us. I remember very little of those early years, except for vague sensory memories of being cold and hungry, and of rats running across my chest, though it's possible those were merely dreams.

Most of what happened to us during the six years of World War II came to me in the form of stories told to me by my mother, a gifted storyteller blessed with an excellent memory and remarkable patience, who nightly sent me off to sleep with her favorite tales, which I never tired of hearing. One story in particular was told to me so many times that I came to believe I actually remembered it.

It was 1942, and the war in Europe was raging on all fronts. The fact that Romania was a German ally turned out to be a double-edged sword for its Jewish population. At first there was hesitation to surrender the Jews, who were well-assimilated members of Romanian society, for deportation to the extermination camps. But as German occupation solidified its grip on the nation, Romanian cooperation with the Nazis became routine. Pogrom-like beatings, round-ups, and killings of Jews became daily occurrences. The ruthless Black Guard, an elite unit of the Romanian army with a particular penchant for Jewish persecution, was apparently given carte blanche to roam the streets, beating and murdering Jews at will.

One cold and gloomy winter morning, a squad of Black Guards set its sights on our apartment building, rounding up a number of Jewish families in the inner courtyard, some fifty or sixty of us. We were then lined up in rows of ten, five or six deep, as several Black Guards set up a heavy machine gun, apparently with the intention of shooting us all. The men were silent, while the women wept quietly. I was in my mother's arms, just under three years old, when I began crying uncontrollably. Perhaps it was hunger or the bitter cold, or simply fear, but this was not a child's mere crying. As my mother told it, my cry was such a strident, ear-piercing shriek that a soldier approached us and ordered her to make me stop. Instead, my screaming only got louder. According to Mama, my wailing was so loud that it caught the attention of a German officer in the street, who proceeded to walk into the courtyard with a platoon of his men and ask the Black Guard sergeant what was going on.

I was still screaming feverishly as the officer walked over to us, looked at me, and touched my cheek. I stopped crying. He told my mother that my blue eyes and rosy cheeks reminded him of his own little boy at home, and walked back to confront the Romanian sergeant, telling him to decamp with his men. An argument ensued, with the Germans holding their rifles at the ready. The Black Guards, visibly angry, packed up their machine gun and walked off in a huff, muttering curses and threats in Romanian. The German officer returned, told us all to go back to our homes, then left with his men.

We stood in silence for a moment, stunned but relieved, not quite believing our good fortune. A small group of people surrounded my mother and me, some crying, some patting me on the head. Old man Wechselblatt, who had been standing in the back, slowly walked over and said to my mother in Yiddish, "*Dus kind hott unz alle geratevet, zein gantz leben vilt ehr gebencht zein.*" This child saved us all, he will be blessed his entire life.

Everyone scattered back to their apartments. That evening, my parents gathered their meager belongings and we fled in the dark, as we would multiple times throughout the war, trying to evade capture and deportation. By the war's end, some six hundred thousand Romanian Jews had been murdered, mostly at Auschwitz, with some perishing at a Romanian extermination camp called Transnistria.

Other memories of the war's early years are distinctly my own. In 1944, when I was about five, we were in the woods when a stray dog bit me in the leg. My father, a jeweler by trade, suspected the dog was rabid. He clasped a razor blade with jewelry pliers and proceeded to make a small fire to heat the razor blade till it was white-hot. He then burned my wound with the white-hot blade. What I remember to this day is not the pain or screaming, but my mother crying while holding me down, and the smell of burning flesh. I still have a large whitish scar on my left shin which looks like an old vaccination mark.

Another memory took place one year later in Bucharest. By then, I was nearly six years old and the war was winding down, the Nazis retreating on all fronts. We were hiding in some basement when we heard the clattering sound of motorized vehicles growing louder and louder, reaching a deafening crescendo. Peering out of the basement window, which allowed a sliver view of the street, we watched in consternation as thousands upon thousands of German troops hurried westward in obvious retreat, looking haggard in their trucks and motorcycles, some running along on foot. The sounds of rumbling tanks, motorized vehicles, and thundering boots lasted for hours and remain in my head still. Then, silence. They were gone. Afraid to move, we remained huddled in the pitch-dark basement for what seemed like eternity, not knowing what would come next.

Suddenly, the rumbling started again. We looked out and saw the Russian troops in their olive green uniforms decorated with red stars and insignia, speeding westward in their trucks, jeeps, tanks, and artillery pieces. None of them were on foot. They looked determined and angry, carrying their Thompson-like submachine guns with round clips. What a sight! The liberators were passing through! The others hiding with us in the basement started cheering, clapping, and hugging. For us, the war was over.

We lived in Bucharest for another three years, narrowly escaping to Paris in 1948 just as the Iron Curtain slammed shut on Eastern Europe, cutting off all access to the west. Our Russian liberators had begun their very own reign of terror.

Chapter Three

Boot Camp

When I arrived at Camp Pendleton outside San Diego on July 19, 1969, everyone was glued to the TV: "One small step for man, one giant leap for mankind..." Neil Armstrong had just stepped on the powdery lunar surface; people all over the world were mesmerized. I too was mesmerized but more importantly, I was tired, hungry, and bewildered. I'd arrived in California with no idea what to expect. I wasn't sure why doctors needed boot camp in the first place. Still, after med school and residency, I figured, how bad could it be?

We numbered approximately fifty men, mostly doctors of various specialties as well as a few dentists, all of us Navy lieutenants. The first evening we were addressed by the commanding officer, Marine colonel Louis Codispoti, a hard-looking, leather-faced man in full dress uniform. Despite the fact that we would soon be assigned to various medical units in South Vietnam, he made it clear that his mission was to train us as Marine combatants; the doctor part was someone else's job. A low murmur rumbled through the room: Would we be facing combat?

"That's right," the colonel informed us. "All personnel assigned to Marine outfits, regardless of rank, medical specialty or physical makeup, need to go through five weeks of Marine Corps basic training. The training will be intense and will cover physical fitness, distance running, steeplechase-type obstacle training, rope climbing, and crawl tactics.

"Military instruction," he continued, "will include assault and defense tactics such as hand-to-hand combat, knife and bayonet training, small and heavy weapons operation, and grenade launching. When you finish your five week training course, I expect you to be Marines, think like Marines, and fight like Marines."

The colonel explained that time was short, which was the reason our training would be especially intense. Five weeks, with one day off every two weeks. When we finally assumed our duties in Vietnam, he told us, we were expected to defend our patients as well as heal them. We were expected to be not only doctors, but soldiers.

"Your training begins at 0530 hours and ends at 1600 hours," the colonel continued. "You will then shave, change, eat dinner, and report to Field Service Medical School at 1700 hours. That is all from me, gentlemen. I now give you Commander Perkins."

Colonel Codispoti walked off, leaving us somewhat stunned, as a stocky, smiling officer in Navy dress blues took his place.

"Now, gentlemen, for the fun part," he began.

"I am Dr. Perkins, responsible for your Field Service Medical School training (FSMS). We will assume that none of you, regardless of whatever surgical skills you may possess, has any experience in the field of combat surgery. We will therefore endeavor to train you in the handling of mass casualties, patient triage, and emergency medicine. You will learn swift and proper patient assessment, evaluation of the unconscious soldier, and treatment of the multiply-injured soldier.

"Your training will include open wound care, surgical care of deep tissues such as bones, muscles, tendons, nerves, and blood vessels. The orthopedic surgeons among you will treat all limb injuries involving fractures with the help of vascular surgery and other subspecialties when needed. The general surgeons will treat all abdominal wounds, neurosurgeons all head wounds, urologists all kidney and bladder injuries, and so on."

Perkins made clear that despite our individual specialties, we would be working in teams, and would be required to assist our colleagues at all times. He also took the opportunity to remind us that

Vietnam is located in Southeast Asia, a tropical paradise blessed with diseases like malaria, typhoid, dengue, and yellow fever, as well as rashes we had never seen before. Perkins explained that his job was to give us a basic understanding of these ailments. We were required to report to FSMS at 1700 hours every day, where we would receive instruction until 2200 hours.

"As a physician myself," Perkins said, "I fully appreciate that this will be for you a somewhat dissociative experience, since you will literally be taught how to kill in the morning and how to heal in the evening. So, you can warn your families in advance that you may all come home next year with split personalities, a little like Jekyll and Hyde!"

Everyone laughed.

That was the last laughter any of us enjoyed for the next five weeks. When reveille (yes, an actual guy with a bugle) sounded promptly at 0500, we jumped out of bed, put on our fatigues, wolfed down a quick breakfast, and assembled in "the square," where we were promptly introduced to Gunnery Sergeant McAvoy, our drill instructor (DI).

This man, who clearly enjoyed torturing people, made every day of those five weeks miserable. He spoke in shouts, with a typical order sounding something like "Get your fucking ass up that hill, SIR!!!" He did not use the word "sir" out of any respect for us, but because as an enlisted man, he was required to address commissioned officers as such. Every morning at 0530, we began the day with thirty minutes of calisthenics and push-ups, followed by a fast five-mile jog in heavy combat boots while carrying forty-pound packs. This was followed by weapons training, which included dismantling and reassembling the Colt .45 semi-automatic pistol as well as the M16 assault rifle, the standard Marine Corps weapon in Vietnam. Target practice followed, after which we were all handed M1 rifles weighing some fifteen pounds and made to run up and down hills yelling "Kill! Kill!"

We were taught how to fix bayonets and charge at mannequins tied to trees, stabbing them repeatedly until they died. We also received instruction in hand-to-hand combat, how to avert a knife attack, how to handle a choke-hold, how to throw opponents, and how to administer fatal blows to various parts of the body. We were shocked to realize how easy it was to kill someone with a single punch or kick to the Adam's apple. Delivered forcefully enough, the blow fractures the thyroid cartilage, shutting down the trachea and causing rapid asphyxiation. Gunny, as Sgt. McAvoy was known, informed us that he had once had to deliver such a blow during hand-to-hand combat in Vietnam. The only thing that disturbed him, he reported, was the crunching sound made by the man's imploding trachea.

The steeplechase course was especially torturous, as it required us to rope-climb up a twelve-foot wall, jump off the top into a sand pit, crawl through metal pipes, run through a tire field, and vault over several pommel horses, all at top speed. If you fell, you were forced to repeat the entire course until you got it right. This was followed by a twenty-minute rest, including a quick lunch of c-rations, which we ate while leaning against a tree.

But without question, the most terrifying part of our entire training was the crawl-under-live-machine-gun-fire. Imagine a hundred-yard flat stretch of dirt with wood partitions six feet apart, a little like a swim meet, but with a barbed wire ceiling two feet off the ground. We were required to low crawl as fast as we could while cradling our M1 rifles in our bent elbows, peering out from under our helmets to make sure we were going straight. Behind us was the *tat-tat-tat-tat-tat* of machine gun fire. This was no mere simulation; several machine guns, located behind the starting line, were firing live rounds just above the barbed wire.

If you panicked and stood up, you would be hit by the live rounds. If you lagged behind, a megaphone-wielding Gunny would scream, "Move! Move! Move! Get your fucking ass going, sir!" Those hundred yards felt like a hundred miles, during which some of us gave up our lunch. The back of my neck ached, my arms burned from carrying that miserable rifle, my elbows were scraped raw, and the entire front of my body was chafed from the endless crawl through the dirt.

When it was over, I felt a strange sense of accomplishment mixed with terror. But there was no time to reflect on my feelings. After the crawl-under-fire came another five-mile run. Finally, 1600 arrived. Blisters, aches, and sores aside, I felt relieved the day was over. Then it was back to the barracks for a quick shower, change, and dinner, this time of real, welcome food.

Compared to boot camp, Field Service Medical School was a delight. Not only did it offer civilized relief from boot camp's physical rigors, we were given extensive instruction in all forms of combat surgery, emergency medicine, and treatment of tropical diseases. My civilian training as a surgeon in New York City had taught me nothing about treating multiple gunshot wounds, traumatic landmine amputations, or mass casualties. I had arrived with virtually no knowledge of triage science; now suddenly I was getting a crash course in the basic principles of wartime medicine.

I was intrigued to learn that fresh wounds in Vietnam were almost never closed the same day. Instead they were treated with so-called delayed primary suturing (DPS). It had become apparent soon into the war that most wounds were caused by high velocity objects like shrapnel fragments, which inflicted severe soft tissue damage and deep burns that were not readily apparent. If the wound was merely cleaned and the skin closed immediately, the damaged and dead tissue would fester, causing a wound infection that would require further surgery. The doctors soon learned they were better advised to first clean the wound and simply cover it with sterile dressings, then go back the next day and remove any additional dead tissue. On a third look, if there was no more dead tissue and the wound appeared healthy, the skin could then be closed for DPS.

Using this procedure, the majority of wounds remained clean, avoided infection, and needed no further surgery. That was a valuable lesson learned in the early and mid-'60s by our Vietnam combat surgeons, who imparted it to us.

With regard to orthopedics, we were taught strict general principles, mainly that major open limb fractures suffered in combat should be cleaned, closed and splinted, rather than fixed with metal devices to prevent infection. Permanent fixation could be done later, either on a Navy hospital ship offshore or at a rear echelon hospital in the Philippines or Japan. The principal exception to that rule was a combination fracture and vascular injury, where vascular repair or grafting was required in order to save the limb. In such cases, the orthopedic team would first achieve solid metallic fixation of the fracture. This would provide a stable construct for the vascular repair, which was fragile at best and could not survive in an environment where jagged bone fragments were moving around. If the metallic fixation became infected, that problem could be addressed later, but at least the limb was saved. This kind of instruction was most informative to us civilian surgeons, because combination orthopedic-vascular injuries were rather rare back home.

On my first day off, I contacted a friend who lived in nearby San Diego. I had met Frieda Heller on a trip to Israel earlier that year. Always gracious, Frieda invited me to spend the day with her, and proceeded to show me the town, taking me to her favorite restaurants, and lavishing me with a hospitality that was a welcome relief from Camp Pendleton.

The five weeks of boot camp were surreal, a combination of the exhausting, the exhilarating, and the bizarre. Our last day was capped by our official promotion to the rank of Lieutenant Commander and the receipt of our individual orders for assignment in Vietnam. Little did I suspect how useful the attempt to transform us into soldier-surgeons would be.

Chapter Four

Welcome to Vietnam

On August 24, 1969, I was placed on a flight to Danang, via Honolulu and Tokyo, together with my old pal and fellow orthopedic surgeon Dick Nottingham, affectionately nicknamed "Sheriff." Dick and I first met as freshmen at Columbia College in 1956, only one year after my family had emigrated from France. We were both pre-med and upon graduation, we were both accepted to New York Medical College, where we each took an early interest in orthopedic surgery.

We even attended the same orthopedic residency program at the Hospital for Joint Diseases in New York City. Not only did we train together for five years, we both became commissioned officers in the US Navy under the Berry Plan. Now, having suffered through boot camp together, we were on our way to the same Marine Corps hospital outside Danang.

When we arrived at First Medical Battalion on the evening of August 26, the hospital compound was under attack by the Vietcong (VC). The Marine Sergeant who had picked us up at Danang airport and driven us the forty-five minutes to First Med led us in a low crouch to Hootch 8, our assigned lodging. Machine gun fire could be heard up close at the perimeter of the compound, from both Vietcong and Marine units. Smoke and explosions from grenades and VC rockets could not only be seen and heard but also smelled, the air pungent and dusty. After dropping our duffle bags on the plywood floor, Sheriff and I low-crawled to the far end of the darkened hootch and lowered ourselves into the bunker, where we were hastily introduced to our hootchmates, whose faces were illuminated by flashlight.

"Nice reception, guys," I said. "The place always this friendly?"

"Every night," replied Dave Whitney with a smile, "or worse. But hey, look at the bright side: You never get used to it! So…welcome to Nam!"

There were laughs all around, and chatting in the dark.

After about an hour, the attack was over, and we climbed back into the hootch, lights back on. The six bunks were all occupied. In addition to Dave Whitney, there was Bob Widmeyer, Roger Crumley, and Tom Kilroy. We were all orthopedic surgeons except Crumley, who was ENT. I immediately liked my hootchmates, who seemed like a friendly, rowdy bunch.

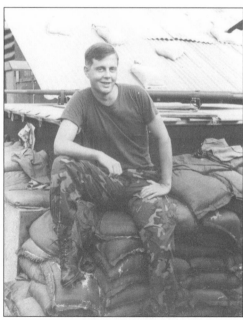

Dave Whitney outside Hootch 8

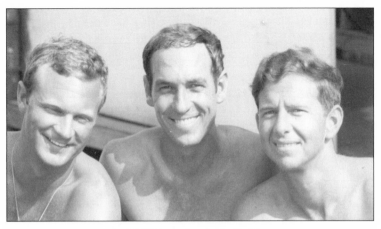

L to R: Bob Widmeyer, Roger Crumley, Tom Kilroy

Each bunk was flanked by a small set of drawers into which Sheriff and I crammed our meager belongings. I lay down on my bunk, hands behind my head and thought, "I made it, I'm here…now the hourglass starts running."

The following morning at 0700, we reported to the commanding officer with our orders. Captain Jim Lea, "the Skipper," was a tall, handsome man with penetrating brown eyes, an engaging smile, and a firm handshake. A skilled internist and hematologist, he also impressed me as thoroughly honest. Indeed, as we would learn in the coming months, he treated all of his fellow soldiers with respect, whether they were career officers like him or reservists like most of us doctor draftees. Captain Lea demanded strict adherence to duty and protocol. At the same time, he could often be found hanging around the OR, looking in on difficult cases, day or night, to show support for his staff.

As we stood before him, he quickly explained our duties. We would be on call every day from 0600 to 1800 for the treatment of incoming casualties. Every third night, we'd be assigned night duty in teams of two. Each of us was responsible for running the orthopedic clinic one afternoon a week, and we also got one day off a week.

We soon learned that the Skipper was an interesting man who enjoyed a good time. He often hung out with us evenings, drinking beer, chewing the fat, and laughing it up. He also had a girlfriend, the supposedly stun-ning Anneliese Hoenlein, herself the commanding officer of the *Bremer-haven*, a German hospital ship docked offshore, where sick and injured Vietnamese civilians received free treatment.

On his days off, Captain Lea would disappear and not return until early the next morning. We all knew where he had gone. Still, we didn't discuss it among ourselves out of deference to the Skipper. The only joke going around was that he was the world's only naval officer with allegiance to two navies.

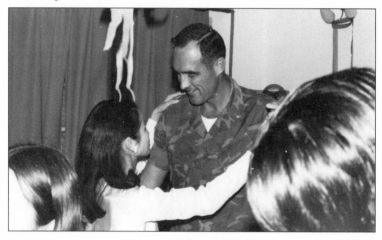

Lea dancing with a Vietnamese interpreter

Some time before my arrival in Vietnam, Hootch 8 had acquired a reputation for rowdiness. For whatever reason, the hootch had long attracted reservist types like myself, who unlike the career military offi-cers, were irreverent and somewhat undisciplined characters, a little like Hawkeye Pierce and Trapper John in MASH. We laughed a lot, drank beer, partied, and liked to poke fun at "lifers," as career types were called.

I quickly realized that my year in Nam would be more tolerable than expected. Yes, I'd been sent to a war zone, but at least I had the good fortune of landing in Hootch 8. I thought of something my father often said in Yiddish: *auch mit pech darf min huben glick.* (Even with bad luck you need to be lucky.)

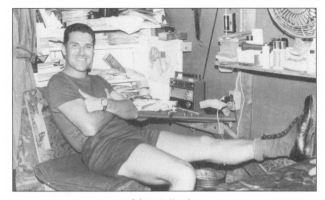

Relaxing in Hootch 8

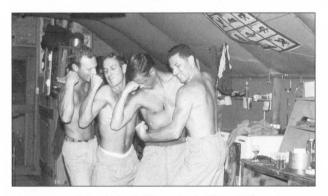

Flexing with (L to R) Widmeyer, Crumley, Whitney, Brief

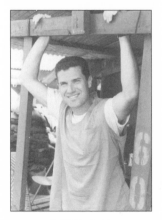

Outside the Hootch

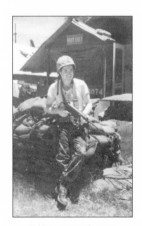

Holding a captured weapon

Chapter Five

The Action Starts

The action began promptly the next morning as the squawkbox woke me with a raspy "Dr. Brief to ER, Dr. Brief to ER STAT!" Having been advised to sleep in scrubs, I jumped into my "jungle boots" and jogged over to the ER-triage area. A wounded Marine was lying on a litter, his fatigues cut off, his legs covered with multiple wounds. Some were large and gaping, oozing blood, while others were small, almost pinpoint. A Navy corpsman was hosing down the soldier's legs to wash off the field dirt and mud.

"Frag?" I asked.

"Yes, sir," nodded the corpsman.

Fragmentation grenades could propel literally hundreds of fragments at high velocity, inflicting massive damage to soft tissue, severing blood vessels, and breaking bones.

"X-rays?" I asked.

"Over here, sir."

Corpsman Radcliffe pointed to the view box on the wall, which showed there was shrapnel from groin to ankle in both legs and a fractured right fibula. Luckily, there were no fragments inside the knee joints.

"Check the abdomen?" I asked.

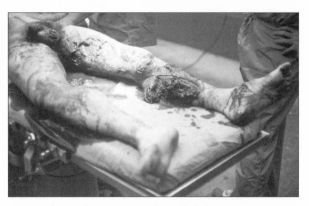

Fragmentation grenade wound to both legs.

"Yes sir, looks clean."

"Recent food?"

"No, sir. Lucky, no breakfast."

"OK, let's take him in. Anesthesia here?"

"Waiting in OR, sir."

The OR, one of six, was large and well lit. A medium height, handsome Filipino man with an engaging smile came over and extended his hand.

"Sonny Alafriz, anesthesia. I checked him out in triage, he's good to go."

We flipped our masks over our faces and as the scrub tech transferred the patient to the OR table and hung up both legs on IV poles for sterile prep, I went to the sink outside the door to scrub up.

When I walked back into the OR, the patient was asleep, draped and ready to go, with tourniquets in place at the upper thighs. I gowned and gloved quickly and went to work, wound by wound. With the large ones, some of which were 5×5 inches, I excised the burned skin edges, removed all the dirt and shrapnel I could find, and cut away dead muscle.

Living muscle tissue twitches and retracts when you cut it, so I had to slice away all the dead muscle until I reached living, moving tissue. I also had to be careful not to accidentally cut into a nerve or blood vessel lurking underneath. As I trimmed, Radcliffe, who was sharp and fast, cauterized any bleeding vessels.

In FSMS we'd been taught that, as opposed to civilian surgical incisions, which are carefully planned to safeguard important structures, war wounds occurred randomly, with no regard for anatomy. Small entry wounds were left alone. Large wounds were sterile dressed after cleansing, then covered and bandaged to be re-explored the following day. If they were clean, the skin was sutured. If more dead tissue and dirt were found, it was back to the OR the next day, until delayed primary suturing became feasible. And so it went for up to a week.

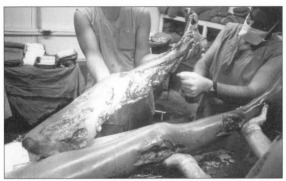

Wounds all cleaned up – for OR the next day

It took me ninety minutes to do both legs, a bit slow I thought. I knew I would need to work faster if I was to keep up with the high casualty volume. I had five more cases that day and seven the next. Every one of my five orthopedic colleagues had a similar case load. Still, I quickly began to gain confidence and improve my working speed. I thought to myself that this wasn't all that bad. But I was wrong.

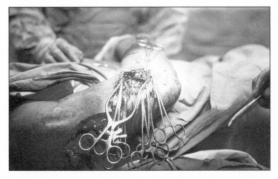

Gunshot wound to the arm. Radial nerve damage calls for extensive reconstruction later

Chapter Six

Twice the Heartbreak

On my third day, I was awakened at 0545 by ear-splitting, hootch-rattling chopper noise, which was soon followed by a message from the squawkbox, "Dr. Brief to ER STAT, double amp!"

Double amp? I ran to triage and there he was, my first double amputee. The grunt, who could not have been more than twenty years old, was lying there emitting a low, plaintive moan. He had tourniquets on both sides just below the groin, and both his legs were gone at mid-thigh. His stumps were singed, black, and ragged, with strands of hanging muscle and tendon. On the right side, jagged femur bone protruded some four inches, oozing blood. His genitals appeared mangled, unrecognizable. I felt physically ill. Nothing in my medical training, not even FSMS, had prepared me for this.

As soon as corpsman Radcliffe had hosed down his stumps, we took the poor guy to the OR and I got to work. I excised the burned skin edges and cut away as much dead muscle and shredded tendon tissue as I could. I found the femoral artery and ligated it shut, then identified the femoral and sciatic nerves, cutting them neatly across. I had to saw off the femur high up and round off the end for later prosthetic fitting.

I was astonished to find a couple of screws deep inside the soft tissue and also some foul smelling, greenish-brown stuff...

"Radcliffe, is this what I think ..."

"Yes, sir, water buffalo shit."

"Goddamn sonofabitches," I muttered. "How could they do this?"

After about an hour of irrigating, trimming, and snipping, we had both stumps cleaned and dressed. Then we called for urology to take over. We planned a return trip to the OR next day, for more cleaning and excision of dead tissue before shipping the GI out to the *Sanctuary,* our offshore hospital ship.

I felt wiped out, angry, and depressed. I believe I aged a whole year that day. Little did I suspect that treating double amps was to become an almost daily routine. Hundreds of cases, one after the other, day and night, more of them than we cared to count, more of them than we could stand.

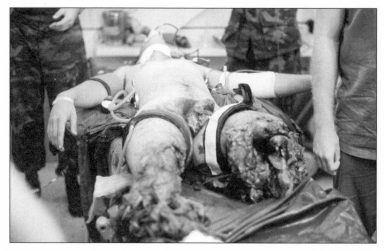

Double amputee

How did this come to be? From the outset of the war in the early '60s it was clear that U.S. forces controlled the country during the day, while the enemy, or Charlie, ruled at night. The enemy consisted of the North Vietnamese Army (NVA) regulars, and the Vietcong (VC), who were South Vietnamese guerilla fighters on the communist side. Ho

Chi Minh, the legendary North Vietnamese leader who had defeated and expelled the French in 1954, controlled everything from his central command in Hanoi.

Among other strokes of tactical genius, our military leaders came up with the following plan: Since the enemy operated mainly at night, why not send out pre-dawn patrols to search, surprise, and destroy them? After a few months of relative success, these search-and-destroy missions, operating along well-established jungle paths, became obvious to the enemy. In the thick of night, the vc would lay down a type of Claymore mine, also called a booby trap or "Bouncing Betty." These homemade explosives, at once primitive and deadly, were typically made of coffee cans stuffed with plastic explosives, rocks, screws, bolts, and assorted garbage such as water buffalo feces. The whole thing was buried a couple inches below the surface, with the detonator rigged to a spring-loaded device. When a soldier's boot, usually belonging to the "point man" (the first soldier in a single-file platoon), tripped the device, the bomb did not detonate right away but rather jumped two feet out of the ground before going off, taking one or both of the point man's legs with it and wounding one or two men behind him.

Day in and day out, time after agonizing time, the routine remained the same. Of the nearly two hundred amputees I personally treated in Nam, some single but mostly double, 167 of them were point men.

In my sixth month in-country, out of sheer anger and desperation, I wrote the following letter to General Patrick McWilliams, Commanding Officer of the First Marine Division, with the Skipper's approval.

> *Dear General,*
>
> *I am one of six orthopedic surgeons serving at 1st Medical Battalion. It has come to our attention that devastating double amputee injuries are brought in to us with sickening and alarming regularity. These injuries, which occur during pre-dawn search-and-destroy jungle patrols, are usually caused by underground explosive devices, and most commonly affect the platoon point man. Is there anything that could be done from a military tactical viewpoint to modify, cur-*

tail or somehow redirect these patrols in an attempt to rectify this dreadful situation?

We are extremely upset and distraught over this, since our principal mission as doctors in Vietnam is to save life and limb. All, especially our Marines, would appreciate anything you could do to rectify this dire situation.

Very truly yours,

Lieutenant Commander L. Paul Brief, (MC), USNR

February 15, 1970

I never received a reply. Of course, it's possible my letter never reached the general, as all mail was censored. Meanwhile, the patrols continued unchanged and the casualties kept rolling in. Later, I would learn that many of the amputees we took in ended up amputated one level higher back home because of sheer soft tissue damage and infection. So that BKA patients often ended up AKA, lower thigh ended up upper thigh, and upper thigh ended up as hip disarticulations.

Not only did the double amputee nightmare follow me home, it haunted my dreams for decades.

Chapter Seven

Mosquitoes, Small Ants, and Other Creatures

A few weeks after my arrival at First Med, I got the bright idea to start jogging for physical fitness. But where to jog? Leaving the hospital compound was forbidden, so I decided to do laps around the helicopter landing zone (LZ), a large square area covered with thick metal plating to accommodate the heavy chopper traffic. All went well for several weeks until one late afternoon when I was running laps, going over the day's cases in my mind.

Although aware that the area was heavily infested with mosquitoes, I wasn't overly concerned about malaria, as we were all required to take a weekly prophylactic dose of chloroquine-primaquine, also known as the CP pill. Every Sunday after breakfast, under Sergeant Major Roberson's watchful eye, we took the pill, affectionately known as "Ho Chi Minh's revenge" because it gave us the runs until Thursday.

So here I was jogging along as the sun was going down and dusk began to blanket the area. "Damn," I thought, "these mosquitoes sure sound loud today." Then, suddenly, I became simultaneously aware of several facts. First, I was jogging around the LZ, which is always watched by the enemy. Second, I was wearing a white t-shirt at dusk, and third, those were not mosquitoes but sniper bullets whizzing past me!

"You stupid jerk," I thought to myself, "they're shooting at you!" and took a flying dive into the ditch that surrounded the LZ. Lying as low as possible, I pulled off my white t-shirt and threw it as far as I could. Then I lay there half naked waiting for the dark.

When darkness finally fell a good ninety minutes later, I ran back to Hootch 8 in a low crouch. "Hey, Brief, where have you been?" my hootchmates wanted to know. Then Whitney said, "Wow, look at your back! What are those?"

It turned out my entire back, neck, arms, and legs were covered with hundreds of mosquito bites. By morning I was feverish. The itching was so intense I had to go to sickbay, where I was given a shot of cortisone, along with some antihistamine pills, antibiotics, and aspirin. The fever took two days to break. I considered myself fortunate that I did not come down with malaria. That Sunday, I asked for a double dose of the CP pill, never mind Mr. Minh's revenge. That was the end of my jogging.

But mosquitoes were not the only form of enemy insects in Vietnam: there were also the small ants. These hateful, minuscule creatures were everywhere. Small enough to crawl through the screen walls of our hootch, they got into our clothes, our beds, and our belongings. They'd bite, too, leaving tiny red marks that itched.

Exasperated, I developed a routine where I would stand just outside our hootch door each night and exclaim at the top of my lungs:

"God, please, I beg you, no more small ants!!! Give me large ants I can see and fight! These small ants are driving me crazy, they're everywhere. I can't stand them anymore, so please, Lord, help me and enlarge my ants…NO MORE SMALL ANTS, PLEASE!!"

The laughter from my hootchmates and neighbors only encouraged my wailing, and so I developed various versions of my lamentation.

"God!!"

Prolonged silence.

"Small ants are no longer driving me crazy! I *am* crazy! It's over! They've driven me over the edge! PLEASE GOD, I beg you, give me large ants and allow me to regain some semblance of sanity! AAAAAAAAAAAAGH!!!"

I even attempted to bargain with Him.

"Please, God, I'll do anything! I'll become more religious, I'll even study to be a rabbi! But I beg You, no more SMALL ANTS! They're the devil, I tell You, the devil himself, and they'll be the death of me! Please, magnify them, do SOMETHING to help me…PLEEEEEASE!"

But the Almighty never heeded my supplications, and the ants remained. As for my colleagues, who at first seemed to good-naturedly tolerate my ranting and raving, they took revenge by dubbing me "Small Ants Brief," a moniker which stuck.

Scorpions were much easier to see, if more frightening, with a sharp stinger atop their curled-up tails. We took to turning over and shaking out our jungle boots before pulling them on, and occasionally a small scorpion would scurry away and vanish into some dark hootch recess, although I cannot remember any one of us ever suffering a scorpion bite.

But unquestionably, the most fascinating wild creature in Vietnam was the "fuck you lizard." This animal, most likely a kind of gecko, was active only after dark. Our battalion dentist, who was in possession of all kinds of weird military equipment, claimed to have staked out the lizard and spotted him, using his night vision goggles. On quiet nights, as we sat around talking, we'd hear a sudden, piercing "*uck-yoooo…uck-yoooo…uck-yoooo,*" whence the creature's name. People from other hootches would quietly walk over and sit listening to the bizarre chant that usually went on uninterrupted for several minutes. On occasion, the squawkbox would intone quietly: "Attention, fuck you lizard working out by Hootch 10," at which we would all slip over to hear the familiar tune.

When I returned home, I made an attempt to find the name of the lizard, but I was never able to find any listing or description of such an animal. Still, I heard its song with my own ears, as did all my hootchmates and colleagues at First Med, a song forever imprinted in our memory.

Chapter Eight

White Elephant

The White Elephant was a military bar and hangout in Danang, where we would occasionally go to have drinks, listen to music, and pass the time with other Americans from surrounding military units. It was a large, noisy, cheerful place, and my first visit there was a memorable one.

I arrived one evening when I was off duty, wearing newly washed jungle fatigues, a starched cap, and shiny boots. At the entrance was a large sign that read: "No weapons beyond this point!" So I unbuckled the gun belt holstering my .45 semi-automatic and hung it on a hook next to the others. When I stepped into the noisy saloon, I was greeted with loud rings from a large bell hanging over the corner of the bar, the bell rope being pulled repeatedly by the bartender. All heads turned to me, laughing, clapping, and cheering. I turned to look behind me, thinking maybe they were welcoming some dignitary who had followed me in.

But no, it was definitely me they were cheering. With a start, I realized what had happened – I had walked into the bar wearing my cap. Apparently, there was an old military custom they never told me about in boot camp: Any man walking into a military bar wearing a "cover" is required to buy the entire house a drink! This oversight is traditionally heralded by the bartender to the delight of all present. Even though it was happy hour and all drinks were fifty cents, I had to shell out about sixty bucks, given that the joint was packed. Smiling but embarrassed, I threw my cap on the table where Whitney, Crumley, and Kilroy stood up to cheer me and pat my back.

We talked and joked about how I'd never make that mistake again. Then Crumley whispered to me to look over to the far corner table. It was occupied by a large group of men and women in civilian clothing, except for Captain Lea, who was dressed in his jungle fatigues. Next to him sat a striking blonde woman who spoke animatedly as everyone around her smiled and listened.

"That's Dr. Hoenlein," said Crumley. "The German hospital ship's chief doctor. Isn't she something?"

She was stunning. Who could blame the Skipper for disappearing on his day off and not coming back until the next morning?

As we got acquainted with the other officers, exchanging stories and experiences, we had a few drinks but remained sober; none of us were especially heavy drinkers. When it came time to leave, Whitney, Crumley, Kilroy, and I packed into a motor pool jeep driven by a Marine corporal, and headed back towards First Med. Fifteen minutes later, about half way to our destination, our vehicle came under small arms fire from the thick vegetation across the road. The corporal expertly drove the jeep into a shallow roadside ditch and we all rolled out of the vehicle. Taking cover in the ditch, we turned and faced the road. We pulled out our weapons and returned fire, the Marine blasting his M16 and the four of us aiming our .45s toward the enemy fire, which we could still see and hear from across the road. It was the typical "ack-ack-ack-ack" of the AK47 assault rifle, slower but louder than the M16.

Bullets flew all around, making their typical buzzing sound. One struck the jeep windshield, shattering it. I reloaded twice, emptying all three clips, firing toward the enemy and keeping my head as low as I could. We were lucky the ambush was staged from only one side of the road. A two-sided ambush would have prevented us from ditching the jeep, putting us in serious danger. We were also fortunate that no mortars or RPGs were launched, as we had none to return fire with.

After about fifteen minutes, the firing stopped and we waited in silence. None of us had been hit. When all was quiet, we crawled back into the jeep and, keeping our lights off, drove away into the night as fast as we could. It was a dark night but we could see fairly well, as we'd all become adapted to night vision. We arrived back at First Med feeling fortunate. I actually felt good about our handling of the situation. We'd been ambushed, but we didn't panic, and promptly returned fire. By the time we got back to the base, we were shaken but unhurt.

The next morning, a Marine platoon patrolling the vicinity of the ambush discovered the body of a young man identified as a VC, apparently dead of gunshot wounds to the head and chest. Was he one of our attackers? We never found out, but for the rest of the year, Whitney, Crumley, Kilroy, and I teased one another, each of us claiming the hit, although we knew full well that if indeed the VC had died in the attack, he had most likely been killed by the corporal's M16, a much more powerful and accurate weapon than our .45 semi-automatics.

After that night, whenever we left First Med for any destination, we brought along our M16s in addition to our .45s, and wore helmets and flack jackets too.

And I never again walked into a military bar wearing a hat.

Chapter Nine

RPG

On the morning of September 24, 1969, we were awakened by unusually frantic chopper traffic, soon followed at 0615 by an ominous announcement over the squawbox: "Attention, Attention ortho team: all members report to the Skipper's office STAT! Attention, Attention ortho team!"

This had to be bad news as we'd never heard such a message before. Whitney, Widmeyer, Kilroy, Gregersen, Nottingham, and I hustled over in double time, and assembled nervously before the Skipper.

"Gentlemen," he began, "we have a dire situation and not much time. A grunt has just been medevaced here with a live M79 grenade embedded in his thigh. Here, see for yourselves."

He put up a 14×17 x-ray plate on the viewbox behind his desk. There it was, as several of us whistled in amazement. The rifle propelled grenade (RPG) was sitting in the inner thigh, intact, right next to the femur. I'd never seen or imagined anything like this. A live grenade inside a man's thigh? It was potentially catastrophic.

"Needless to say, we've got to go in there and retrieve it," the Skipper said.

"Commander Dave Lewis is on first trauma call and is setting up the OR. The patient is getting a spinal anesthesia as we speak. Now let me get right to the point and explain why you're all here. Lewis is all set to go ahead with this case, but I've given it some thought and I don't want him to do it. He doesn't know that yet. You see, Lewis is going home next week, and at this point I think it's unfair to expose him to such danger. He's been here a whole year, he's stressed out, and he deserves to go home. All other general surgeons are busy in the OR and since ortho is on second trauma call, I've decided one of you should handle this."

We all threw furtive glances at one another.

"Now I don't want any volunteers, and I believe the only fair way to do this is to draw lots. I'll pick one of your names out of a hat, but know this: I can't have a guy in there with that live M79 if he's going to be scared to death and cause a disaster. So if I pick your name and you think you're just not up to it, let me know and I'll pick someone else. No hard feelings. Understood?"

With that, he proceeded to write out our names on six slips of paper, crumpled them up, and threw them into his hat. We stood in stunned silence. I was thinking of a similar incident that had taken place at a Saigon Army hospital a year earlier. The grenade had detonated in the OR, killing doctor, patient, and anesthesiologist. As the Skipper mixed the papers up and picked one, I'll never forget the sweat running down my back into my scrub pants and the feeling of raw terror in my heart. I'd never known such fear before, not from school bullies, sniper bullets, Vietcong rockets, or roadside ambushes.

Then he uncrumpled the paper and read the name.

"Brief."

I couldn't believe my ears. My knees buckled a little and the sweat poured down harder. The grenade was going to blow and I was going to die. Images flashed before me, of a young naval officer knocking on my mother's door, holding a folded flag, a sad-looking Jewish chaplain at his side. Mama opens the door, cries out, and falls to the floor.

"Well, Brief," said the Skipper, "what's it going to be, yes or no?"

All eyes turned to me as thoughts went through my mind with lightning speed. What was I going to do? My name had come up fair and square. Was I up to the task? What if I declined, and another guy went in and got blown up? Could I live with the guilt?

The Skipper was about to speak again when the door flew open and Lewis came running in.

"All set, Skipper," he said, red-faced. "Sandbags are up, patient's ready, spinal is in. I'm going in!"

"Just a second, Lewis, just hold your horses a bit here! You're NOT going in! You're rotating out of here in a few days, you've done your job, you've got a wife and kids back home, and I've just picked Brief here for the job." The Skipper stood up and added: "And that's an order."

Without a second's hesitation, Lewis replied calmly but firmly:

"Skipper, I'm on first call, the grunt came in on my watch, this is MY job. I'll be damned if I'll put someone else in harm's way just because I'm going home soon. Now if you feel you have to write me up for disobeying an order, go right ahead, but I'm going in."

With that, he rushed off and we watched through the screen as he walked into the OR.

Again, we stood in stony silence. Whitney, behind me, put his hand on my shoulder. Then, without another word, we all filed out, including the Skipper, and walked to the OR, where a small crowd had already formed. Nobody spoke.

After a couple of minutes, I turned around and was shocked to see the gathering crowd: doctors, corpsmen, chopper pilots, Marines in full combat gear, patients in bandages and pajamas, in wheelchairs, on crutches, patients holding up injured buddies. There must have been over four hundred men there.

We waited in the sun, dreading the awful explosion that would mean death for Lewis and his patient, and spell heartbreak for all of us.

I felt relief, mixed with guilt and concern for Lewis. There had been no time to answer the Skipper's question, but my mind was still buzzing with it. What would I have said, yes or no? It was a moot point now: the die had been cast. I was not a religious man but found myself praying silently for Dave Lewis's safety and that of his patient. I repeated my prayer over and over in silence, with closed eyes and a heavy heart.

After an hour that felt like ten, we heard the OR door being kicked hard from inside. Skipper went to open it, and there stood Lewis in his surgical gown, cap, and mask, with the M79 in his bloody, gloved hands.

We started to applaud, but the Skipper turned and motioned for us to be quiet. Gunnery Sergeant Donnellan from the bomb squad walked up, hoisting a large sand-filled box, into which Lewis slowly deposited the grenade. Captain Lea closed the OR door and we instinctively filed out behind Gunny Donnellan, heading for the steep perimeter drop-off a short distance away. We gathered at the brink and stood with baited breath as Gunny threw the heavy box as far as he could, all eyes watching it sail down about two hundred feet, violently exploding on the rocks below.

It was the loudest sound I have ever heard. Not the explosion, but the simultaneous outburst of delirious joy, relief, and victory that came from our four hundred chests. We were jumping up and down, hugging the Skipper, hugging Gunny, hugging one another. It was the happiest moment of the year, like all the holidays wrapped into one. Somehow, we had snatched a victory over the misery of war, over the danger and carnage all around us, over death itself.

For his extraordinary heroism, Lieutenant Commander David H. Lewis was awarded the Navy Cross. The injured grunt got a Purple Heart and a trip home. And I got something also. I got to wonder for the rest of my life whether or not I would have had the courage of a Lewis, had he obeyed the Skipper's order and stepped aside. Would I have gone in there, knowingly facing death, or would I have opted out? Would I have been too scared to do it or would I have been capable of overcoming my fear? Did I, or did I not, have the guts?

I have stayed awake nights pondering the possibilities and asking myself these questions, questions to which I'll never know the answers.

Chapter Ten

Scared in Retrospect

That evening Hootch 8 held a party for Dave Lewis, a combination hail-to-the-hero and farewell bash, as he would be returning home the following week. We cleaned up the place as best we could, put up makeshift decorations, and planned for a real feast. We had beer, booze, the works, even some wine, and recruited our very own culinary expert in the form of LCDR Bob Cave, a general surgeon who looked like Elton John and cooked like Jacques Pepin. He worked all afternoon preparing his signature dishes: sliced marinated steak, grilled stuffed chicken, garlic mashed potatoes, almandine vegetables, and a fancy salad.

I too prepared a dish (the only dish I knew), a mushroom ragout with polenta, learned from my mother. Crumley set up the music, playing cassettes of The Beatles, The Rolling Stones, and The Who. He also played several Hootch 8 "anthems," including "Born to Be Wild" by Steppenwolf and "People Are Strange" by The Doors.

Everyone was invited, and the place was packed. We took turns crowding around Lewis, asking him again and again to recount his story, minute by minute. He patiently answered our questions, expressing puzzlement at what a big fuss was being made over the whole thing. When he took the "foreign object" out of the Marine's leg, he insisted, he had simply been doing his job.

But Lewis also told us a few things that night we hadn't previously been aware of. When the Marine was first medevaced in and Lewis rushed to examine him, the Skipper had Lewis's blood drawn and cross-matched in the event that he was injured and needed a transfusion. The Skipper also had an adjacent OR fully set up in case the grenade detonated and Lewis became a patient himself.

"I suppose it was during all these preparations that the Skipper had a change of heart and decided he didn't want me to tackle the job. But my mind was made up. So what if I was getting out of here next week? Fair is fair. I was on first call and that was that. Imagine, just imagine, if I'd complied with his order and another man had gone in and gotten blown up. How could I have lived with the guilt? Naah, that grenade had my name on it, and I was damned well going to remove it, or die trying."

We sat shaking our heads in admiration as he continued.

"One funny aside, though. When I walked into the OR with the soldier lying on the table and sandbags set up all around him, it was immediately clear to me that the sandbag wall on the side I was to stand on was much too high for me. You see, the Skipper had the wall set up for a guy about six foot three like himself, forgetting for a moment that I was only five foot seven!"

We all laughed, attracting the attention of the Skipper a short distance away, who soon walked over to us.

"Skipper," said Lewis with a smile, "your sandbag wall was set up for a much taller man. Thank you though, for having such a high opinion of me!"

There was laughter and applause all around as the Skipper replied: "Lewis, you insubordinate rascal, you do indeed stand tall, taller than any of us."

Later that night I approached Lewis myself.

"Say, Dave, be honest. Were you scared? I'll admit I was scared to death when the Skipper picked my name out of his hat. How about you?"

"You know, it's funny," he replied, "I literally had no time to be scared. Things moved so fast, the excitement was so high, what with all the adrenaline, that I just went ahead and did what I had to do without thinking too much.

"But once I handed off the grenade and started closing up the wound, I heard the explosion about five minutes later. Then it suddenly hit me what danger I'd been exposed to. So I started sweating profusely and my hands shook a lot. Yeah, I guess I was scared. Scared in retrospect."

Chapter Eleven

Heavy Casualties

Lewis's departure on October 4 coincided with a significant increase in casualty volume. A constant traffic of medevac choppers dropped off their dreaded loads day and night. Amputees, including double and sometimes triple amputees, in addition to all types of multiply-injured soldiers continued to pour in, as gut-wrenching as ever. The men on call were overwhelmed and required assistance across surgical fields to handle the load. We worked all day and most nights. There was little time for sleep and we were all exhausted.

One day in mid-December, we got a general call of "full alert," which meant all surgeons had to report to triage at once. A large personnel-carrying truck had gone over a powerful mine. The thirty-eight Marines standing in the truck were blown twenty feet into the air before the truck came crashing down in flames. Although five Marines had miraculously escaped serious injury, ten were killed immediately, including the driver and shotgun rider, with twenty-three severely wounded. They were brought to us in three choppers, as medical personnel swarmed the ER.

The injuries were indescribable: mangled limbs; arms and legs shattered to pieces; skulls fractured; spines crushed; ribs and pelvises broken; chests caved in. It was a scene the likes of which I'd never seen before.

Some of the x-rays looked straight out of hell. Because the massive impact came from below, the boys' limbs and bones had been propelled upward with unimaginable force. We stood there in shock, looking at x-rays of tibias projected up into the pelvis and femurs crashed through the pelvis into the abdomen, but the most surreal were the cases in which intact femur bones had telescoped straight through the abdomen up into the chest; the x-rays showed the femur resting vertically right next to the heart. I had the fleeting thought that perhaps this was some twisted nightmare, but no such luck. It was all too real.

We went to work in teams of two or three, trying to pull limbs downward and relocate joints. But as we soon found out from the soldiers' otherworldly screams, we first had to put them to sleep. We set up each of the six ORs with two or three litters, taking the worst cases in first, each of our six anesthesiologists handling two, sometimes three cases at a time. Some of the poor devils needed their chest and abdomen cracked open simultaneously to disengage their telescoped bones. One of the Marines, whose femur had lodged itself all the way up in his right lung, died on the table. During an attempt to pull the bone down from his chest, a jagged fragment from his splintered femur veered sideways and pierced his heart.

We worked non-stop for four days, scuttling between OR, recovery, and triage. Some of the boys needed to go back to the OR repeatedly to stop their bleeding and address their various injuries. Most needed multiple transfusions. We soon ran out of blood, and all First Med personnel – including doctors, corpsmen, Marines, and yes, even lightly injured grunts – were made to donate pints. As a relatively rare B-negative blood type, I was still asked to donate, even though I had just given blood ten days before, which only added to my state of exhaustion.

After some ninety-six hours, the nightmare finally began to stabilize. We took turns sleeping in four-hour shifts, returning to work for eight hours, then sleeping again for a couple hours.

Sadly, we lost two boys, the one mentioned above and another who died of massive hemorrhaging from his chest and lacerated liver. In spite of the surgeons' tireless efforts and multiple transfusions, the

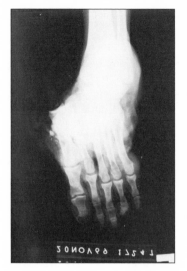

Top view: Severe fracture-dislocation of foot

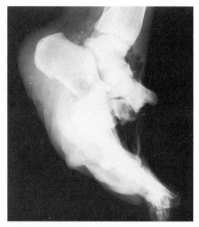

Side view: impaired blood supply

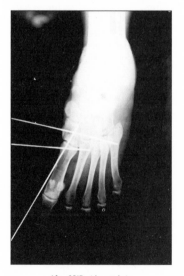

After ORIF with metal pins

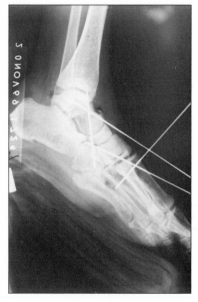

Side view: foot was saved

bleeding could not be controlled. The poor soldier lapsed into irreversible shock and died two days later. We all felt miserable, exhausted, and depressed.

Once stabilized, all injured survivors were choppered out to the USS *Sanctuary* for further treatment. From there, they were transported to Japan, before their final transfer to a naval hospital back home.

Then the monsoon came, with its gale-force winds and torrential rains, which made it impossible to see anything further than six feet away. As the weather was still hot, we could actually shower in the rain. We would strip naked, run out and get wet, then hop back under the hootch's overhang, where we would soap up, then dash back out to rinse off. The whole thing took about three minutes.

Everything was wet, soaked through from the downpour and the dampness. Nothing stayed dry. We wrapped cameras, weapons, medications, and electronics in heavy plastic bags, sometimes using body bags from the hospital's "graves" department, which was dedicated to caring for fallen soldiers and their remains. The only good thing about the monsoon was that it stopped the war cold. Who can fight when you can't see? After three solid weeks, the rains stopped and the war resumed.

Each of us in orthopedics took turns covering the walk-in clinic or "sick bay," where grunts from the bush wandered in with problems ranging from malaria to exhaustion, from trench foot to achy muscles to various sprains. Mostly, they just wanted a few moments to talk to someone, to vent, to stop fighting, to interrupt the maddening routine of patrols, ambushes, raids, and rocket fire, of watching their buddies get maimed or killed. There were many days when I felt more like a psychiatrist than an orthopedist.

One day, a black Marine some twenty-five years old limped in, complaining of an injured ankle. Upon examination, it seemed to be a rather minor sprain. When I asked him what happened, he said:

"Walking on patrol early morning still kinda dark all of a sudden on the right comes *tat-tat-tat-tat-tat-tat-tat-tat-tat-tat*... mothafucking ambush! Shit, we all hit the deck, returned fire to the right, low-crawl toward the fire, y'always crawl toward the fire in an ambush. Goddamn grenade land next to me, grab it and throw it back, scared shitless...Then sarge in front of me catch a round right in the chest, yells out then, 'lay there still!' 'Sarge! Sarge!' I shake him, he don't move, then I scream, 'Corpsman! Corpsman!' He crawl over and says, 'sarge dead.' Cocksucker dead! More fire now on left *tat-tat-tat-tat-tat-tat-tat-tat-tat-tat*...We all crawling backward now to try to get away, look like a double ambush. I'm sweatin, scared shit firing my weapon and sarge's weapon toward Charlie. Behind me two guys set up the mortar and blast'em *pow-pow-pow-pow-pow* five or six in a row to right and left. M60 man also fire like crazy, shift his weapon right, left, right, left, back and forth. Noise is fucking crazy man, crazy. We hear Charlie yell, more mortar rounds *pow-pow-pow-pow-pow*. Then like silence, man, nothing. We wait quiet. Ambush over. We lose sarge and three grunts, even my buddy Sam. Then chopper come, pick us up."

He talked like that for over twenty minutes, as though in a trance, reliving an endless nightmare. He was obviously cracking under the strain and needed a break. Although he only needed an Ace bandage, I decided to put him in a walking cast and crutches for a whole week, just to give him a chance to catch his breath before going back into combat. I called up our psychiatrist Harold Fischer, who agreed to see him and maybe add on a couple extra days of rest.

Then, as I was putting on his cast, he told me possibly the strangest thing I was to hear my entire year in Nam.

"Doc, gotta tell you something. It's a secret, man."

"Then why tell me if it's a secret?"

"Gotta tell somebody, just gotta. My secret."

"Go ahead, I'm listening," I said, applying another roll of plaster.

"Doc, I'm a convict, fifteen years in San Quentin for armed robbery."

"Then what are you doing here?"

"Two years into my sentence they took me out of my cell at night, put me in a small room, man sittin' there in uniform. Man start talking to me and say, 'Son, we givin' you a chance to get outta here. You got thirteen years left so here's the deal: we put you in the Marines, send you to Vietnam on a one-for-five.'

"'What's one-for-five?' I ask and he explain: 'Each year in combat counts as five years in Quentin, get it? So after three years in Nam you a free man.' So I ask, 'Yeah, what if I get shot?' 'That's a risk you take brother,' he say. 'Take it or leave it.' And he stand up.

"So I took it, left that night, didn't tell nobody. Boot camp in Pendleton, then here I am two years already, one to go. I'm a convict, Doc, and you can't tell nobody. They said not to tell nobody. But I had to tell somebody."

"Your story is safe with me," I said. "As a doctor, what happens between me and my patients is confidential and whatever you tell me never leaves this room. So no need to worry."

I finished his cast, fitted him with crutches, then sent him off to the "walking wounded" barracks. I saw him again in the clinic one week later. He was a different man: calm, smiling, rested. As I removed his cast, neither of us spoke. We shook hands in silence and he thanked me and walked off, back to his combat unit.

Over the ensuing months, I casually inquired if any of my colleagues had ever heard anything about convicts being conscripted as Marines. Interestingly, two guys said yes, they had heard the rumors, but had trouble believing them. As for me, I took the man at his word. By the late '6os, the Marines were taking such heavy casualties that they were desperate to beef up their ranks.

Although I had noted the man's name and was aware that a list of fallen Marines was posted every week, for the remainder of my year in Nam, I never checked it. I was afraid of finding his name on it, and I preferred not to know. With time, I forgot his name, and was unable to find it anywhere. But I never stopped thinking about him, and wonder still: Did he survive that third year of combat and return home a free man?

Chapter Twelve

Tokyo Medevac

Although my first five months in-country saw a steady escalation of hostilities and casualties, the final month was by far the most grueling. We worked all day and most nights. The night-time attacks on First Med also escalated, and we soon found ourselves low-crawling into our bunkers four or five nights a week. The ear-splitting chopper rattle was a constant, as was the smell.

Located on an elevated stretch of land, the hospital compound was surrounded by rice paddies stretching out as far as the eye could see. As the practice of "night soil" (using human waste as fertilizer) was still common in Southeast Asia, the entire region reeked of feces. Yet there was another odor just as insufferable, and that was blood. Most of the soldiers who found their way to the OR had blood oozing from every wound, which gave off a fetid, faintly ammoniac stench. Having never been exposed to this much blood in my pre-Vietnam life, I took to wearing double and sometimes triple surgical masks. I was reminded of the old joke about the guy who refuses to become a doctor because he can't stand the sight of blood. For me, it was not the sight of the stuff but the smell of it. I never got used to it.

One morning, Captain Lea sat down next to me at the officers' mess. I never liked breakfast much, so I sat there eating very little, staring at my food.

"Brief, you look morose."

"I'm okay, Skipper."

"No, you're not. I've been watching you, and you're quiet, not your usual jovial self. I think the workload is getting to you, and you're depressed."

"I'm not depressed, and I can still make you laugh," I replied.

"Yeah? Go ahead, tell me a medical joke."

"Guy calls up his doctor and asks how his blood tests came back. Doc says: 'I have good news and bad news. The good news is you've got twenty-four hours left to live.' The guy replies: 'That's the GOOD news?' 'Yeah,' says the doctor, 'The bad news is I wasn't able to reach you yesterday.'"

Skipper laughed and said, "Not bad, now tell me a military joke."

"Okay. Sergeant walks up to the young recruit angry, and says: 'Murphy, I didn't see you in camouflage practice this morning!' The soldier snaps to attention, salutes, and replies, 'Thank you, sir!'"

Skipper cracked up. I thought I'd convinced him, but suddenly he was saying, "Nice try, Brief, but my mind is made up. You need a break badly. So pack your duffle, you're out of here. I'm putting you on the 0800 medevac flight to Yokosuka tomorrow."

Then he walked off.

Those medevac flights were an impressive, weekly phenomenon. Essentially huge transport planes outfitted as hospitals, their purpose was to carry injured troops to rear-echelon hospitals like Yokosuka in Japan, or Clark Air Force base in the Philippines. Lucky for me, the next morning's flight was bound for Yokosuka, located about thirty miles south of Tokyo.

As each flight was required to have a doctor on board in case of emergency, the Skipper would pick one of us each week to hop aboard, then spend a week in the city.

There I was, about three hours into the flight, dozing in my seat, when I felt a tap on my shoulder.

"Doc," said the corpsman, "we need you. Marine in litter twenty-three, his chest tube pulled out, needs a replacement. Come right this way, please."

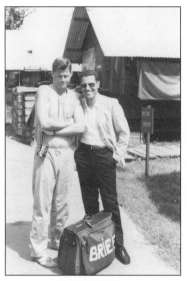

Gary Gregersen wishes he too were going on Medevac

Shit, a chest tube? Why did this stuff happen to me? I hadn't done one of those since my internship ages ago. I followed the corpsman to the soldier's litter and sure enough, his chest tube was out and he was wheezing, his color not too good. Typically, a chest tube is placed into the thoracic cavity between two ribs, then connected to a suction device in order to keep the lung inflated and working. If the chest tube falls out, the lung collapses and the patient develops dyspnea, or labored breathing.

The corpsman had everything prepared: sterile gloves, scalpel, clean tube, local anesthesia, the works. Racking my brain, I found I was able to recall some basic rules about inserting a chest tube: One, the blood vessel runs along each rib on its lower edge, so make your cut along the upper edge of the rib to prevent a hemorrhage. Two, after you make the cut and put the tube in, place a couple stitches on either side of the incision to ensure that the tube won't fall out. Three, if this is a replacement tube, do not be tempted to use the old incision because it'll get infected. Make a new, clean incision one or two ribs higher up.

So far, so good. But for the life of me, I couldn't remember how *deep* I was supposed to put the tube in – three inches, four inches, till I hit resistance? I couldn't remember. It had been too long.

Then I had an idea.

"Corpsman, anyone else on board with a chest tube?

"Yes, sir, two others."

"Good, take me to them."

I grabbed a clean chest tube and went to see the other two GIs. Given that the chest tubes were all standard length, I was able to measure their depth by how much tubing protruded from the men's chests. I put on sterile gloves, and after the corpsman had cleansed and prepped, I chose my spot, injecting a little Novocain as I made the incision and inserted the tube. I pushed it in about five inches, then stitched the incision snugly and taped the tube to the skin. No bleeding so far. We connected the tube to suction, and the soldier's breathing and color began to improve almost immediately.

I felt as though I'd dodged a bullet. Back in my seat, I was unable to doze and instead found myself returning repeatedly to check on my patient. When he saw me, he gave me a smile and a thumbs up, which felt good.

We arrived at Yokosuka in the late afternoon. After all the GIs had been carried off safely, I signed off with the receiving medical officer and hopped the train to Tokyo. Twenty minutes later, I walked into the street and hailed a cab. I was amazed that when the (impeccably clean) taxi screeched to a halt, the rear passenger door opened automatically. I threw in my duffle and said "Sanno Hotel, please." The driver nodded with a brisk "*Hai*" and took off.

The Sanno was a hotel in central Tokyo reserved for US servicemen. Clean, though not fancy, it provided multiple services, including concierge, a restaurant, and a bathhouse. I was booked into a spacious single room where, after checking for small ants, I crashed for a full twelve hours.

The next day I walked around Tokyo enjoying civilian traffic, clean streets, and beautiful parks … with no smells. In the evening I went back to the Sanno and inquired about the bathhouse.

"Ah," smiled the male concierge, "hotsee bath a GI favorite! Should I book one for you?"

"Why not?" I replied.

The concierge made a call and directed me to the bathhouse in the basement, where a smiling Japanese woman wearing a silk kimono was waiting for me.

"Commander, right this way, please."

I was walked along a maze of corridors to a small dressing room where I was told to undress, don a terrycloth robe, and place my valuables in a small locker, dropping the key into my robe pocket. Then I sat in a chair. After a couple minutes, there was a knock on the far door and in walked a tiny, smiling Japanese lady, herself wearing a robe.

"Hotsee bath?" she inquired, and when I nodded, she gestured me through the door into another room, all steamed up, and equipped with a bizarre vertical bathtub and massage table.

Without speaking, she took off my robe and gestured for me to step into the bath, naked, and sit on the built-in ceramic seat. The water was quite hot and after I sat down it reached all the way up to my neck as the tub was built like a gigantic squarish coffee cup. After a few minutes in the steaming water, she gestured me out of the tub and made me stand wearing wooden sandals. Now the tiny bath attendant, who could not have weighed more than eighty-five pounds, proceeded to soap me up from head to toe – everywhere – with thick lathering soap.

She used a natural, rough sponge to scrub my body all over and gestured me back into the tub. All the soap bubbled up to the surface and the hot clear water now felt good. By then I figured I must be the cleanest GI in all of Tokyo. After several relaxing minutes, she gestured me out again, dried me off with thick luxurious towels, and guided me over to the massage table, where she instructed me to lie facedown. She then proceeded to massage me with body oil, before walking on my back, which felt pleasant since she was virtually weightless. Finally, she gestured for me to turn over and began to massage the entire front of my body. After quite a while, she asked with a smile:

"*Szekopp?*"

"What?"

"*Szekopp*," she repeated, and made an unmistakable gesture with her right hand. I understood and nodded yes, to which she added: "Extra yen."

"OK with me," I shrugged, smiling.

But it quickly became clear that she did not know what she was doing. I actually cried out in pain. Seconds later, I leapt off the table, dried-off, dressed, and took my leave.

The next day I slept late, saw a movie in the afternoon, and then figured I would follow the advice of my hootchmate Tom Kilroy. Affectionately known as Killjoy, Thomas Joyner Kilroy from New Orleans was the funniest, most outspoken Southerner I'd ever met and had already been on two Tokyo medevacs.

"Brief," he intoned in his mellifluous Southern drawl, "you goddamn Yankee, listen to me and listen to me good. When in Tokyo y'all jest haul yo'ass over to the Ginza section and find that there Yokohama Lounge, where the ladies love us GI types. Then y'all hook up with one Annie, also known as Yoko, and mention Kilroy."

"Oh yeah?" I said. "What's so great about Annie?"

"What's so great about Annie, mah man, is not only her great body and perfect bosom, but the most amazing lovemaking ah ever did experience in all mah born days. Don't y'all disappoint me now, Brief."

So at about 9 P.M. I went looking for the Yokohama Lounge, which was indeed packed with GIs. But Annie was nowhere to be found, and inquiries with the bartender and hostess were met with shrugs. I sat at the bar nursing a beer, a little dejected at the prospect of a second consecutive bad-luck evening, when a slim, pretty girl sat down next to me.

"You look for Annie?" she asked with a smile.

I guess word had gotten around.

"Yes, I am."

"She my friend, she not here for few days," she continued. "Buy me a drink?"

I gestured to the bartender, who seemed to know her preference and brought her a scotch. She told me her name was Tamiko, but she preferred to be called Ruby. I guess these ladies took on anglicized names to put us GIs at ease. She put her hand on my knee and we talked business. After learning her hourly rate and her all-night rate, all payable in advance, we came to an agreement and hopped a cab back to my room at the Sanno.

We sat on my bed, and I suddenly began to think of the previous evening at the hotsee bath, dreading a repeat performance. Ruby began to undress, but I stopped her. I just couldn't go through with it, and I didn't even know why. She began to cry, which made me feel worse, and I apologized for wasting her evening. Then I paid her the full amount we had agreed upon, which instantly put a stop to her tears. She dressed, and I walked her downstairs and put her in a cab, waving goodbye.

The following evening I was having a late dinner alone at the Sanno restaurant when I noticed a woman sitting by herself a few tables away, writing something and nursing a glass of white wine. Looking at her profile, I could see she was blonde, pretty, about forty years old, and elegantly dressed. Luckily, her table was on the way to the restroom. As I stood up and slowly walked in her direction, I passed behind her and was able to cast a sidelong glance at her writing. She was writing in French, which gave me goose bumps. I continued to the bathroom, washed my hands, combed my hair, then came out and slowly walked back to my table without her seeing me.

Calling the waiter over, I asked him to bring her another glass of whatever she was drinking. He did, pointing toward me as he served her. She turned, lifted her glass slightly, smiled, and went back to her writing.

"Come on, Brief," I said to myself, "don't wimp out." I took my own glass, walked over to her, and said, "*Bonsoir madame, vous permettez que je m'asseye?*"

She glanced up with a smile and a look of surprise, gestured to the chair next to her, and murmured, "*Pourquoi pas… Merci pour le vin.*"

I introduced myself as we continued speaking in French. Her name was Solange Lejeune-Ito. She taught French at a Tokyo private school and was married to a Japanese-American Air Force colonel named Ronald Ito, who apparently traveled a great deal.

I learned that before WWII she had lived with her parents in Vietnam, or "Indochine," as the French called it. In 1939, when she was about ten, her father, a French army officer, was recalled to France to serve in the war. Captured in 1940, he was a POW in Germany until the war's end. Upon his release, he was assigned to the French Embassy in Tokyo as a military liaison officer and moved his family there.

"Fascinating background," I remarked. "You speak all these Asian languages."

"By necessity more than by choice," she replied somewhat sadly.

We chatted in the hotel lounge and I suggested we go up to my room for a drink. She agreed, somewhat to my surprise. We went upstairs and drank some of the scotch I'd brought with me from Nam. Although she seemed genuinely interested, she resisted my advances at first.

Did I harbor any doubts about trying to seduce the wife of a fellow US serviceman? Perhaps, until she confided a few facts about the colonel. First, theirs was apparently a loveless and childless marriage, with no physical contact for the past few years. Second, Colonel Ito enjoyed the company of geisha girls, a fact he made no effort to conceal. Third, Solange told me tearfully that she was beaten on a regular basis. I couldn't believe my ears. This lovely, gentle, educated woman, beaten? Any feelings of culpability I may have had vanished at once. Freed of guilt and fueled partly by the previous night's frustrations, I gently but persistently redoubled my efforts.

We spent the next four days and nights together, catering to each other's deprivation and hunger. The days were spent walking through beautiful Tokyo parks and stores she knew intimately, stopping at quaint restaurants for lunch and dinner. The nights seemed to pass very quickly.

The entire week flew by with dizzying speed, having the elements of a cinematic wartime liaison. It was fast, romantic, illicit, and ultimately doomed. The only thing missing was the music from *Casablanca*. On my last day in Tokyo, we said a sad goodbye. Although we exchanged addresses, we both knew we would never meet again.

When I arrived back in Hootch 8, a little sad but rested and ready to resume working, a grinning Kilroy walked right over.

"Well, mah man, tell me: how was Annie?"

I didn't have the heart to tell him the truth.

"She was great, Killjoy, just great. Everything you said, and more."

Chapter Thirteen

Kaufmann

The months rolled by and men rotated out, replaced by new and interesting characters. I was standing outside Hootch 8 one morning when a fellow walked over, hand outstretched. He was medium height, with dark hair and piercing eyes.

"Hi, I'm Rob, new anesthesia guy," he said, smiling.

"Paul Brief, ortho. Welcome to Nam."

We shook hands.

"Brief with one 'f' or two?"

"Just one, why?"

"Well, my name's Kaufmann with a double 'n', and it's always being misspelled. Pisses me off."

"Really?" I asked. "One 'n' or two, makes such a difference?"

"You bet it does. It's the difference between Christmas and Hanukkah, man."

And like that, I got it. I thought for a second before I replied.

"Actually, Rob, I know exactly how you feel. You see, my name's Brief, German name. But whenever I meet new people, I'm quick to point out that I'm Jewish."

"Why's that?"

"Because God forbid I should be mistaken for some Nazi bastard."

He got it, too. But I instantly regretted my words. "Just kidding, Rob. Welcome to First Med."

He walked off to Hootch 10, his smile gone. Damn, why had I said that? After my childhood in France, you'd think I would have learned to ignore such remarks.

When my family escaped from Romania to France in 1948, anti-Semitism was still rampant across Europe. The kids at school routinely called me *sale Juif*, dirty Jew, which led to daily fist fights. I would often come home with a bloody nose and ripped shirt; my mother was appalled.

"Why do you fight?" she'd ask me. "Just ignore it, *Popol*," she'd say, using the French nickname for Paul. But I couldn't ignore it. I didn't understand why being a Jew set me apart. I looked and behaved much like the other boys, so why did they treat me differently? One classmate in particular took an instant dislike to me, constantly tormenting me with taunts of *sale Juif*.

Jacques Colle was a tall, gaunt bully who mocked me every chance he got, testing how far he could push me. One day during swimming instruction, as I stood at the edge of the pool waiting for class to begin, Jacques, who was already in the water, suddenly yelled out: "Hey, dirty Jew! Don't come into the water, we're trying to keep this pool clean!"

That was it. Without thinking, I took a running start and jumped into the water with all the force I had, striking Jacques in the chest with both my feet. The wind knocked out of him, Jacques fell backward. I quickly slipped behind him and caught him in a neck lock with my left elbow. Then I raised my right hand and raked my nails down his face as hard as I could. He cried out and I pushed his head down into the water with all my strength as he began to gurgle. I held him down with a vengeance and I remember wanting to drown him, to kill him, so he would never call me that name again.

By then, both the swimming instructor and lifeguard had become aware of the trouble, and had jumped in and separated us. They lifted Jacques out of the water and laid him down poolside, where he began to cough and vomit. I saw red marks and blood on his face. The instructor then walked over to me and angrily told me to get dressed and leave at once.

The following morning, I stood before the school principal, Monsieur Vacheron. He was a distinguished, impeccably dressed, middle-aged gentleman with a reputation for being a strict disciplinarian, yet he was kind. Everyone, students and parents alike, loved and respected him.

"Brief, Brief," he said, shaking his head and pronouncing my name "*Bree-eff,*" the French way. I stood before him looking at the floor, my knees shaking.

"What have you done? What's gotten into you? You have consistently been at the top of your class year after year, and now this? Explain yourself."

I said nothing, as tears rolled down my cheeks. He walked around his desk, took my arm and walked to some chairs against the wall, where he sat me down and took a seat next to me.

"*Expliquez-vous, j'attends…*" ("Explain yourself, I'm waiting…")

I told him the whole story: the daily torture of being called a dirty Jew, my puzzlement and despair at being treated differently from the others. I also told him how my father, a jeweler by profession whom the French government had not allowed to work because we were "displaced persons," had been forced to buy and sell goods on the black market to feed our family. I then revealed something my mother had warned me never to divulge to anyone, namely that the previous year my father had been thrown in jail for three months, having been accused of trying to sell a set of stolen silverware. My father, a thoroughly honest man, swore to us repeatedly that he would never have dealt knowingly in stolen goods.

I explained to Mr. Vacheron how Colle had bullied and tormented me for so long that I had simply cracked, taking out all my rage and despair on him. I apologized for my brutality because I did not like to fight, and actually always thought myself a bit of a coward. We sat in silence for a short while.

"Brief, I understand what you've told me, but Colle's parents have lodged a formal complaint and I am obligated to punish you. You are therefore expelled from school."

My heart sank and I slumped forward with my head in my hands.

"For three full days," he continued. "After three days, you will report back to school and exhibit exemplary behavior. One more incident like this means permanent expulsion. Understood?"

I nodded with a mixture of relief and distress. How was I going to explain this to my parents?

Colle returned to class one day after me, his face still bandaged. We never spoke again. In fact, my entire class avoided me and I kept to myself, but not once after that day did I ever hear "*sale Juif*" again. The following year, in 1955, we immigrated to the United States.

I felt regret about my Nazi remark to Rob Kaufmann, and was reminded of a piece of advice my father had given me some years earlier: "Son, every single day of your life, you get at least one perfect opportunity to keep your mouth shut. Don't miss it!"

From then on, there was a coldness between me and Rob for which I felt responsible. Several times, I made overtures to regain his friendship, but he rebuffed them. It would soon become apparent that Kaufmann was a bona fide racist and a bigot, not much different from my old classmate Jacques Colle.

Chapter Fourteen

Mamasan and Other Local Friends

A majority of hootches employed Vietnamese women as housekeepers, addressed with nicknames like "mamasan," "house mouse," and "Nam-mom." Their job consisted of keeping the hootch clean, sweeping the floor, washing and folding laundry, and lending a feminine touch to our lives, as all American personnel at First Med were male. Each housekeeper handled two hootches, and as we each paid her $5 a week plus tips, she could earn about $75 a week, a decent wage in the depressed Vietnamese economy. We had a strict "hands off" policy, as these were all married women, and as far as I knew, we all adhered to the rule.

Cuc was small and pretty, with a ready smile, cheerful disposition, and lovely broken English. She came to work every day at 0800 and left at 1400, walking an hour each way. All Vietnamese walked to and from work, trekking up and down the roadsides all day long, their various wares contained in baskets suspended from thick wooden poles balanced across their shoulders. They tended to walk in a bouncing gait, a learned technique meant to lighten the weight of their loads. As we drove by on our jeeps, we watched in amazement as they glided along with seemingly effortless grace. Though slight of build, they appeared able to carry heavy cargo almost acrobatically, their sandaled feet barely touching the ground.

While we all liked Cuc, for a time she seemed unable to master her job. When she left in the afternoon, she took our laundry with her. She washed it in the river, hung it out to dry, then folded it in the early morning and brought it back in two huge baskets. The problem was, she seemed to have no idea which laundry belonged to whom. Inevitably, every evening was a mad scramble to recoup our respective stuff. Labeling our laundry with markers didn't work, as Cuc apparently couldn't read the names. In the morning she'd just place a neat and totally arbitrary pile of laundry on each of our beds. A few of us would take turns sorting out the mess, running between Hootch 8 and 9 to deliver laundry to the proper owners in what we called the "laundry express." It would have been a real nuisance if it weren't so funny, with a bunch of us running back and forth like characters in an old Keystone Kops silent film, delivering laundry to our friends like mail from home.

Cuc took a lot of time off, each time leaving us a note with an excuse that might have been convincing were it not so often repeated – usually, a dead relative. This happened so frequently that Roger Crumley took to saying that Cuc must have eight grandmothers and fourteen aunts who are all Vietcong, because they're dropping like flies! One letter in particular was so blatantly fabricated that I entered it into "The Hootch 8 Scriptures," a compendium of miscellaneous absurdities which more or less became my responsibility.

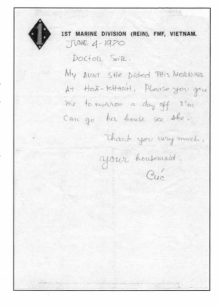

The morning after her "loss," she would show up cheerful as ever. After all, how bad could the loss of one aunt be when you have an endless supply of them?

Cuc liked to talk to us about her family, but mostly she complained about her youngest son, Tranh.

"Tranh problem, he no listen. *Bookoo* trouble, he run everywhere. He fourteen years old, act like eighteen with fighting. Always I worry about Tranh."

On a rainy morning in March 1970 I was called to triage and there was Cuc, sitting and crying. Next to her was Tranh, crying quietly while lying on a gurney with a mangled right hand. Tranh wasn't just trouble. He was Vietcong, and had tried to set an explosive charge under an American officer's jeep. The plastique had detonated prematurely, and he was lucky to be alive. But his right hand was severely damaged, with his pinky finger blown away, and his ring finger having suffered multiple and severe open fractures.

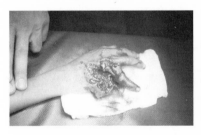 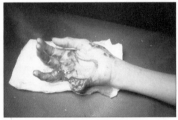

Tranh's hand, palm down   Tranh's hand, palm up

I took him to the OR at once, washed and cleansed his wounds, controlled the bleeding, then applied a sterile bandage to the hand. The following morning, all wounds seemed clean, so I went ahead with a "fillet procedure" on his ring finger. Hopelessly damaged because of the multiple complex fractures, the entire finger would serve as a vascularized pedicle flap graft to cover the gaping wound left by his amputated pinky. I therefore removed the ring finger's bony skeleton, cutting out every jagged bone fragment I could see or feel. I took care to identify and preserve all blood vessels and nerves. Then I used the entire flap to cover the gap and trimmed any excess skin to obtain a perfect fit. Finally,

I secured the flap with nylon sutures and was able to give him a functional, if imperfect, three-finger hand. After a number of weeks, he was fully healed and seemed able to write again.

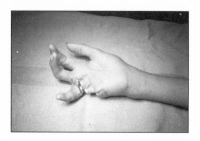

Next day, palm up

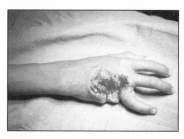

Next day, palm down

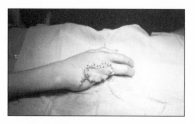

Fillet graft completed

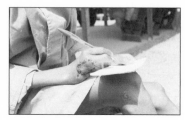

Holding a pencil

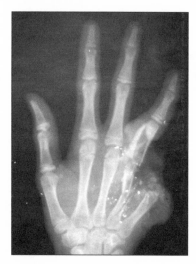

Tranh's x-ray before surgery

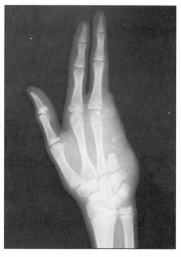

X-ray following reconstruction

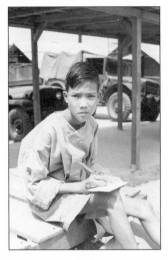

Tranh

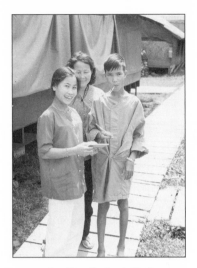

Cuc with son Tranh and a friend

Cuc never asked for another day off after that. Instead, she whispered to me daily how thankful she was that I had fixed her son's hand. In a casual discussion with the Skipper, I asked whether we should fire Cuc for being the mother of a Vietcong.

"What the hell," Skipper said, "these VC are all around us anyway."

Cuc stayed, and as if by miracle, each of us started receiving his own laundry every day.

LCDR Sonny Alafriz, our Filipino chief anesthesiologist, was an extremely well trained and skillful doctor who could administer anesthesia in any form to any soldier at any time. Regardless of how agitated, uncooperative, multiply-injured, or grime-covered an incoming grunt might be, Sonny would swiftly take over and have the soldier ready for surgery in record time. Whether general, local, spinal or nerve block anesthesia was required, he would swoop down on the patient with his team, quickly cut away clothing, clean the required areas, and swiftly administer the anesthesia. Never in civilian practice, either before or after Vietnam, have I seen an anesthesiologist with such precision and speed.

In fact, Dr. Alafriz took it upon himself to teach all us orthopods how to quickly and safely administer spinal anesthesia. The logic behind this was that during times of mass casualties, when the anesthesia team was overwhelmed, the orthopods could handle some of the lower extremity injuries ourselves. Alafriz would bring us into the OR individually or in groups of two, and show us the anatomy and the proper location for spinal needle insertion. Then he demonstrated the technique for spinal tap and introduction of the medication. After a couple of sessions, I felt confident I could perform the procedure myself. Ultimately, I would put in over one hundred spinal anesthesias in my year at First

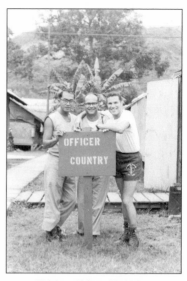

With Sonny Alafriz and Paul Rubino

Med, sometimes two or three in one day, as did the other orthopods.

Together with our Filipino neurosurgeon Dr. Nicodemus and a couple of Filipino corpsmen, Sonny Alafriz had a small band. Sonny played piano, Nicodemus played sax, and one corpsman played trumpet. Together with Crumley's guitar and my harmonica, we would sometimes play with them in the evenings in an attempt to dampen the boredom.

But the Filipino tradition that stood out was the pig roast. Every month or so, Alafriz and Nicodemus would travel to the local convent where pigs were raised, and bring back a pink, plump *cochon*, as the locals called it, which was French for pig. Then the entire Filipino team would dig a large pit in the back near the weightlifting setup, slaughter the pig and set up fire, spit, and crank. The roasting would go on for hours, with people taking turns stoking the fire and turning the crank. The flames, the roasting pig, and the gathered men made quite a spectacle, especially at night. Because of my Jewish background, I declined to partake of the meat, but I enjoyed the scene and often helped carve and serve the various morsels.

Then there were the Koreans. South Korea, a staunchly anti-communist United States ally, sent troops over to fight on our side. And fearsome fighters they were. Republic of Korea marines, or ROK marines as we called them, were known to be super tough. Tall and athletic, these elite troops all seemed to be martial arts experts, and on occasion we would travel over to their barracks a couple of miles north of us to watch them practice and demonstrate their judo and jiu-jitsu skills. Strictly regimented, they were loyal and obedient soldiers who never questioned orders. Superbly trained, they were ruthless in combat and took no prisoners. All the NVA and VC troops they encountered in the field were killed outright, no questions asked, no mercy.

When ROK marines suffered casualties, they were medevaced to First Med to be cared for by their own fully staffed medical team. In appreciation for their alliance, we allowed them the use of our hospital facilities, equipment, and supplies, while they provided the manpower to care for their wounded.

Given that Colonel Kang was the only orthopedic surgeon on their staff, we would sometimes assist him on difficult cases. A tall, powerful man with skillful hands and a ready smile, Kang spoke decent English, as he had received some orthopedic training in Seattle. But in the OR he was all business, yelling staccato orders in Korean to the scrub tech, circulating nurse, and anesthesiologist. He even yelled at the patients.

On one occasion we were working together on a case in which a ROK marine had suffered extensive wounds to his lower extremities. We both worked hard, cleansing the wounds and trimming away damaged tissue, Kang on the right leg and me on the left. Suddenly the soldier started moaning out loud, his anesthesia obviously not working. Kang looked at me and said "Spinal not working!" then started yelling at the anesthesiologist, who injected more medication and tried to calm the soldier down. But the moaning grew louder and suddenly Kang was screaming at the patient to shut up. To no avail, as the poor devil was by that point screaming in pain. I watched in amazement as Kang grabbed a large Richardson metal retractor, tore down the drape in front, and began banging the soldier in the head repeatedly with the retractor.

I yelled, "Kang, stop! What are you doing?!!" and tried to grab his arm. But by then he was screaming at the top of his lungs, hitting the soldier over the head again and again.

It worked. The soldier went silent, and Kang stopped yelling, throwing the Richardson on the floor with a loud clang. We both resumed working as if nothing had happened. Nobody spoke. We finished the case and I left, very upset.

The following questions occurred to me: Had the soldier stopped yelling because the anesthesiologist had put him under? Had he gone silent just so Kang would stop hitting him? Or had he been knocked unconscious by repeated blows to the head?

I never found out. But I did stop in the recovery room the next morning, and there was Kang's patient, awake and alert and drinking tea, with both legs heavily bandaged. He also had a big bandage on his head. I stood at his bedside, smiled at him and asked, "Okay?" He nodded, smiled, and gave me a thumbs up. Those ROK marines really *were* tough. As for Colonel Kang, we never discussed the incident. But from that day on, whenever I worked with him, I made sure to get to the OR first, where I would remove the Richardson retractors from the surgical setup and hide them with the complicity of the scrub tech.

We soon discovered there was something sad and disturbing about our Korean allies. While their marines suffered similar casualties to ours, mainly bullet and shrapnel wounds, burns, and amputations, the Koreans' attitude toward the amputee problem was disturbing. In those years, Korean society suffered from a bizarre intolerance of amputees. Upon their return home, these poor devils were ostracized and stigmatized. Their own families considered them a burden, a source of shame and embarrassment. Painfully aware of the dismal fate that awaited them, these unfortunate ROK marine amputees, from the moment they arrived at First Med, begged and pleaded to be put to death.

Every waking moment, from the time they came out of anesthesia, all they asked for was to die. They refused to eat, tore at their bandages, and maintained a constant wailing refrain of "please kill me!" in Korean. Kept alive by intravenous feeding, they would pull their IV tubing out again and again in hopes of starving to death. The Korean doctors and orderlies who cared for them agonized over this; the entire situation was unbearably painful to witness. These poor men, unable to face the grim prospect of returning home in their damaged condition, really and truly wished for death.

Over the course of my year in Nam, three of these Korean amputees were found dead in their beds without apparent reason. Had they hoarded pain pills and taken them all at once? Were these assisted suicides with the help of some ROK marine buddy? Or did some Korean doctors participate in acts of euthanasia? These questions remain tragically unanswered.

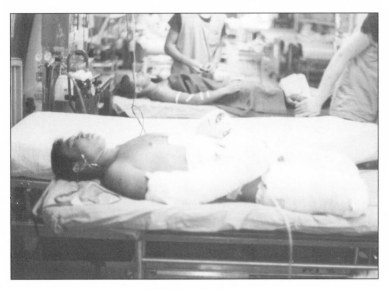

ROK Marine double amputee

Chapter Fifteen

Buddies

Roger Crumley, ENT/plastic surgeon-in-training, was a jovial, witty, mischievous guy, who, in my opinion, was largely responsible for the rowdy reputation enjoyed by Hootch 8. He organized our beer parties, picked the rock music we listened to, and even, at one point, convinced us to form a singing group he dubbed "The Hootch 8 Lifers," an ironic reference to our distaste for "lifer-think."

We harmonized in hearty if mediocre renditions of "Proud Mary," "Old Man River," and "Yellow Bird," all of them sounding much better after our audience had enjoyed a few beers. But Crumley's true forte was the practical joke. When Paul Rubino, a kindhearted, well-trained, but somewhat naïve general surgeon from Chicago arrived in Nam and landed in Hootch 8, Crumley went right to work on him, dragging me along.

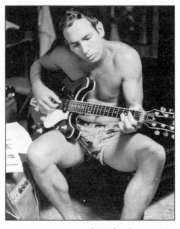

Roger Crumley strumming

How could anyone help liking a Midwest-born and -raised surgeon who spoke with a heavy Italian accent? Especially one who was gullible, recently married, and lovesick? He even referred to his beloved wife back home as "Mamma."

One evening soon after Rubino's arrival, we were sitting around laughing and talking when Crumley discreetly pulled me aside and said: "Brief, I'm going over to triage to make an announcement. You stay here and make sure Rubino hears it." A couple minutes later, the squawkbox intoned:

"Attention! Attention! We have an urgent need for an Italian-speaking surgeon in triage! Attention! Attention!"

Rubino shot up from his seat, said "That'sa me!" and took off for the ER. Shortly afterwards, he walked back through the door arm-in-arm with Crumley, both laughing hard. We all stood up and cheered: "Welcome to Vietnam, Paul!"

"How could I fall for this?" laughed Rubino. "An Italian-speaking surgeon needed in Vietnam? It must've been the beer!"

Rubino was very good at his work, extremely conscientious, and seemingly tireless, but his naïveté was boundless. On my next trip to the PX, I picked up a couple bottles of a popular Italian wine called Ruffino Chianti. After we drank it, I soaked off one of the labels, cut out the name "Ruffino," backed it with cardboard, then pasted it onto a standard size plastic nameplate. I walked over to Paul and told him I had a gift for him. He looked at the nameplate and calmly announced:

"My name issa Rubino, not Ruffino."

"Close enough," I replied. "Look at the nice blue background."

"Sorry, it's notta my name."

"Rubino, Ruffino, what the hell's the difference, Paul? I worked hard to make this thing, and now you won't wear it?"

Sensing I was disappointed, Rubino agreed to pin it to his t-shirt, then with raised forefinger, added seriously:

"But only insida da 'ootch!"

He wore it for weeks, all of us complimenting him on his handsome new nameplate. I knew he was only doing it so as not to hurt my feelings, like the truly good soul that he was.

A few weeks after his arrival, Rubino expressed interest in acquiring an underwater camera, as he and his new bride enjoyed snorkeling and were considering scuba diving. On our next trip to the Danang PX, Crumley and I brought him along and he purchased a late model Nikonos, an underwater camera manufactured by Nikon. He studied the manual and played with his camera for weeks, saying: "I can't wait till my wife Angela sees this! *Che bella cosa!*"

Soon afterwards Crumley approached me with an idea, and we sat down to talk to Rubino.

"You know, Paul," said Crumley, "you should be aware of a very important piece of information about your Nikonos that's not in the manual."

"Oh?" replied an intrigued Rubino. "What's that?"

"Well," continued Roger, "a friend of mine, a diving instructor back home, owns a Nikonos camera like yours, and I clearly remember him saying that this type of camera must be kept underwater at all times."

"Huh? That's interesting," replied Rubino, "because the manual makes no mention of that."

"Yeah, well, these instruction manuals are full of mistakes, Paul. Besides, it's an underwater camera and if it's kept out of water, the seals may dry up and crack, then water could leak in when you go diving."

"Wow, that's amazing! What do you think, Brief?"

"I agree with Roger," I added with a twinge of guilt. "I've heard the same thing. It makes sense to keep it submerged."

"Okay," sighed Rubino. "Let's do it."

All three of us went to triage, picked up a plastic bucket, half-filled it with clean water, then went back to Hootch 8 and gently placed the camera at the bottom of the bucket.

"You see," said Crumley encouragingly, "not a single bubble. That means the seals are all perfect, and now they'll stay that way!"

About two weeks went by until we could wait no longer. When we finally came clean and admitted to Rubino it was all a prank, he was a little miffed at first, but his good nature soon took over and the entire hootch had a good laugh over some beers.

Several months after his arrival at First Med, Rubino began to notice that the ringing in his ears, something many of us experienced due to the constant chopper noise, was accompanied by hearing loss. He got tested at the nearby Air Force base, where they found a slight hearing loss, gave him earplugs and earphones to wear, and instructed him to return in six weeks. Unfortunately, the new tests apparently showed such rapid deterioration in his hearing that it was recommended he be sent home for reassignment to a less noisy environment.

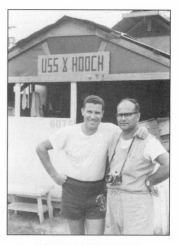

Rubino sports his Nikonos camera

We had grown quite attached to Rubino and were upset to see him go, so we planned a big farewell party on the eve of his departure. About a week before his scheduled flight home, Paul had gone to the PX and ordered a few custom-made suits and sport coats from the local Hong Kong tailor. He had already had two fittings a couple days apart. On the day of his party, he went to pick up his new clothes, then came back to Hootch 8, excited to try everything on as we all watched.

But when he put on one of his new suit jackets, he promptly announced: "I can't raise my *harms*."

"What?"

"Look at my jacket, I can't raise my *harms*!"

Sure enough, both suits and sport coats had the same problem. The armpits had been sewn too low or too tight. We called the PX, but it was too late; the tailor had left for the day and Paul's flight was scheduled for 0800 the following morning. We did our best to console him by trying to convince him that his suits were beautiful, and anyway he didn't need to raise his "*harms*."

"Look, Paul," said Crumley seriously, "back in Chicago, when you need to hail a cab, let Mamma raise her *harm*, you don't need to do it. And besides, your tailor back home can fix this with no problem."

Unconvinced, Rubino gave us no choice but to cheer him up by getting him good and drunk at his farewell party. Actually, we all felt good that in this particular case, none of us were at fault. In the morning, we got him up and walked him to the airport-bound shuttle vehicle, all of us sad to see him go.

Bob Widmeyer, orthopedic surgeon and frequent "hootch commander," was known for his weightlifting, his calmness under fire, and a coolness which earned him the name "Leatherman." A certain tall, corpulent, and middle-aged NCO named Chief Collins liked hanging around our little outdoor weightlifting setup located in a small clearing behind the hootches. Obviously impressed with Widmeyer's strength and lifting ability, Collins frequently mentioned he'd liked to arm wrestle him. Widmeyer politely declined at first, then became annoyed.

"Collins, please get off my back. I've no desire to arm wrestle you."

"What's the problem, Commander, are you chickenshit?"

"No, it's just that I don't arm wrestle old men."

"Why, Commander," replied a vexed Collins, "this old man will take you down in an instant. You *are* chickenshit, aren't you?"

"No, I'm not. I just know that if we do it, you'll get chest pains and have a heart attack. Not that I give a shit. So just buzz off and leave me alone."

The bickering went back and forth but Collins would not relent. When Widmeyer finally gave in, and proceeded to take him down within three seconds, Collins turned beet red and clutched his chest. Widmeyer stood up and calmly said, "Don't say I didn't warn you," and walked away. That was the end of the arm wrestling challenge, and the birth of Leatherman. We rushed Collins to the ER, where the cardiogram came back normal, as his chest pains were most likely muscular.

Widmeyer was not the only avid weightlifter among us; pumping iron had become a favorite pastime for fending off boredom, much like in stateside prisons. Among the aficionados was one Bill Miller, a member of Hootch 12, also dubbed "Phuc Dup Hootch." Hootch 12 was home to various characters like Lockhart, Bardenheier, and Blaylock. Jim Lockhart, general surgeon, had a heart of gold and ended up working with me on multiple occasions. Thoracic surgeon Joe Bardenheier, whose dark undereye circles we attributed to a combination of insomnia and grumpiness, grew corn behind his hootch. LTJG Howard Blaylock was a quiet, somewhat hapless, hospital administrator type who kept a pet duck.

Bill Miller liked his beer, so one night when he went missing, his hootchmates alerted us and we all went out looking for him. We finally found him on the bench press, barely breathing, unable to lift the two hundred and fifty-pound barbell off his chest. His skin was nearly blue.

It turned out Miller had consumed an enormous amount of beer, then gone lifting on his own. With no one around to spot him, he'd been unable to lift the load off his chest and collapsed. We quickly hoisted the weight off him and took him to the ER, where he was put on oxygen, after which we brought him back to "Phuc Dup Hootch" to sleep it off. From then on, we kept a vigilant eye on Miller, making sure he did not go pumping iron alone again. Imagine dying in Vietnam not from a Vietcong bullet, but from asphyxiation caused by bench-pressing while intoxicated.

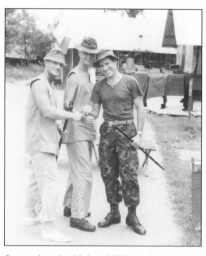

Bumpety-bump handshake with Widmeyer (L) and Whitney®

Chapter Sixteen

The Lieutenant's Induction

Dave Whitney, an orthopedic surgeon and the most veteran Hootch 8 resident, was a gifted storyteller whose dry delivery often left us in stitches. But while he told his stories in deadpan monotone, he was nearly as mischievous as Crumley. Whitney had recently returned from a short trip to Sydney, Australia, where officers were often sent to get some R and R.

"So we get off the plane in Sydney," intoned Dave in his slow, Jack Benny style, "and these jokers gather all US military personnel in a large classroom-type hall, where a uniformed Aussie customs officer addresses us. 'Gentlemen, welcome to Australia.' Yeah well, for starters, you wanna welcome us to Australia, don't pack us all in a cramped room like cattle. Then he continues his welcome speech. 'Please be aware there are four principal types of goods which are strictly banned from import into this country, as follows:

1. Weaponry of any type, strictly banned.
2. Any type of alcohol, banned.

3. Any drugs and drug paraphernalia such as pills, capsules, powder, marijuana, hashish, injectables, syringes, needles, etc...banned.
4. Pornography of any kind, shape or form, banned.'"

Speaking in an impeccable Australian accent, Whitney continued: "'But gentlemen, before your luggage is thoroughly searched for any of the above and to spare you an unpleasant journey to the Sydney Central Constabulary, you will be given the opportunity to discard any and all banned materials yourselves. Your luggage is presently in a large hall next door. There, you will be granted fifteen minutes of full private amnesty time to discard any banned materials in specially provided containers. After that, you may proceed to customs, where your luggage *will* be meticulously searched. And be warned, gentlemen, as our officers are quite thorough and our penalties quite stiff. That is all and again, welcome to Australia.'"

Little did we suspect that Whitney's theatrics would soon prove quite useful to us.

Shortly after Paul Rubino's departure, one Lt. Reginald Parker, our new xo, arrived. Lieutenant Parker wasn't just career Navy, he was an Annapolis graduate and the quintessential lifer. As xo, his job was equivalent to that of a civilian hospital administrator, which meant Parker carried a good deal of authority. It soon became clear he intended to exercise every bit of it. Within forty-eight hours of his arrival, he called a meeting of all hospital personnel.

"Gentlemen," he intoned as he stood before us in his crisp, starched jungle fatigues, "My name is Lieutenant Parker, and friends call me Lieutenant. Since my arrival at First Medical Battalion, it has come to my attention that this unit, although its overall performance is up to standard..."

We looked at one another: up to standard? Busting our butts night and day, up to our eyeballs in blood and guts, was that just "up to standard"?

"...has a lack of military discipline, a certain laxity in protocol, which I fully intend to address."

The Skipper, sitting in a chair next to Parker with arms and legs crossed, wore a bemused look on his face, a combination of resignation, amusement, and annoyance. This character was obviously trouble, and had apparently been given a mandate to turn us from a mere hospital into a spit-and-polish showplace of military medicine.

He went on, explaining how we shouldn't spend all our time wearing scrubs, but should instead wear fatigues, starched caps, and shined boots during evenings and days off; how we should be more careful about saluting superior officers who walked by; and on and on ad nauseam. He continued that in the course of his training at stateside facilities, he had become thoroughly familiar with hospital medical protocol, and had noticed that our medical charts and operative reports were lacking detail and polish.

"Oh, yeah, genius?" I thought. Maybe that was because our caseload was so heavy and so grim that we were operating constantly, leaving no time for writing meticulous operative reports. Maybe we were so tired and overworked just patching up the boys that we had precious little energy left to waste on such minutia. Change back and forth into fatigues, walk around saluting people? This joker had to be out of his mind.

"Screw him," said Crumley into my ear. "We'll fix his lifer ass."

"Ah agree," whispered Killjoy behind us. "This prick needs a special First Med welcome."

No so easy. The next weeks were difficult, with Parker seemingly everywhere, inspecting hospital wards, reviewing charts, addressing wounded soldiers like some visiting general, making spot-check visits to ORs and triage areas. We were painfully reminded of hospital administrators back home, some of whom enjoyed making doctors miserable under the guise of upgrading hospital services and improving patient care. Nobody likes to push doctors around more than non-doctor administrative types armed with the authority to do so.

We knew we had to do something drastic. Naturally, it was Whitney who came up with the idea: We would paint the "Lifer Hootch" bright pink. The officers' hootches stood in two neat rows of ten, and were all painted regulation Marine Corps dark olive drab, like pretty much everything else on campus. Hootch 9, across from us, was the "lifer hootch," where most of the career officers bunked, including the overzealous Lieutenant Parker. The Skipper lived in his own private hootch, way at the end.

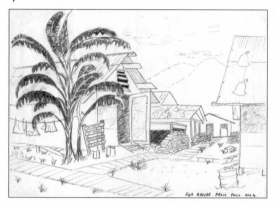

Hootch drawing I sent to my sister Renee

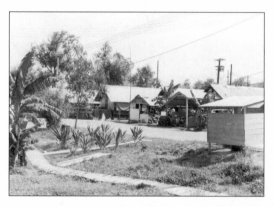

Officer Hootches

On the next free day, Crumley, Whitney, and I drove a motor pool jeep to the Danang PX and acquired several gallons of white and red paint, as well as brushes, rollers, and plastic buckets. On the evening of March 10, we mixed equal parts red and white paint, coming up with a wonderful pink. Then, at 0300 on that warm and moonless night, Whitney, Crumley, Widmeyer, and I slithered noiselessly across to Hootch 9 with buckets and brushes in hand. We went to work quickly and quietly, each of us having been assigned his own area of the hootch.

By 0400, the entire structure except the roof had been painted pink. Allowing the paint some ninety minutes to dry, we then slipped back over, and using red paint and stencils, painted flowers and peace slogans all over the front.

When they awoke later that morning, the lifers were furious. By 0730, Parker had lodged a formal written complaint with the Skipper, openly accusing Hootch 8 of the dirty deed. Skipper pointed out that because there was no proof of the painters' identities, he would ask hootch commanders to appoint volunteers to repaint Hootch 9 as soon as possible. Meanwhile, we all enjoyed the glorious pink color and the sudden tourist attraction status gained by Hootch 9, that symbol of peace in the midst of war, which Marines came to see and photograph from miles around. We also quietly enjoyed the hostile glances of the lifers, who were really pissed.

And so after a delay of about two weeks, a group of us, including Whitney, Widmeyer, and myself, went to work restoring the hootch back to its dreadful olive drab. We had made our point, or so we thought.

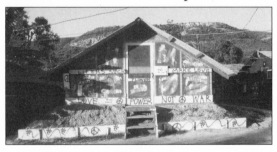

Lifers' Hootch redecorated

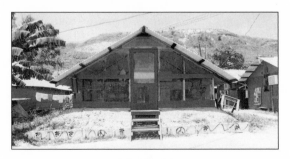

Back to olive drab

In truth, our plan backfired. Parker, now angry on top of being anal retentive, clamped down hard. Rules and regulations reached a fever pitch, with OR and clinic inspections and dress protocol outside the hootches.

We soon learned that Parker was scheduled for his own Sydney R and R four weeks hence, which gave us a little time to plan our next piece of mischief. Using plaster of Paris rolls from the ortho clinic, Crumley, Whitney, and I secretly fabricated a large dildo, first by constructing a plaster framework, over which we layered paper mache. While it was still wet, we molded the paper mache into an anatomically correct model of the male organ, complete with scrotum, bulging veins, and glans penis. After a couple days of drying it in a well-concealed place, we were able to loosen and remove the inner plaster skeleton, and were left with a light yet solid structure. Then we painted it a realistic flesh tone with watercolor paints from the PX, and shellacked it. Over the next couple of weeks, we made discreet, friendly overtures to Parker, who, as we discovered later, assumed we were feeling guilty.

On the evening before his departure to Sydney, Hootch 8 threw a beer party to which we made sure to cordially invite all the lifers. As the party wore on, and the drinking, music, and laughter intensified, the three of us slipped over to an empty Hootch 9. As Roger shone his flashlight, Whitney and I quickly found Parker's duffle on top of his bunk, stenciled "Parker" in large white letters, all packed and ready to go.

Quick as lightning, Whitney jimmied the primitive zipper lock with his penknife and opened the duffle. I then took out two of the neatly folded white t-shirts and carefully wrapped the dildo in them. Placing the package in the center of the duffle, I zipped it back up and secured the lock, the entire operation taking about four minutes. One by one, the three of us calmly rejoined the party, where our brief absence had gone unnoticed. Everyone (especially Parker) was having a grand time.

When Lieutenant Parker returned from his seven days in Sydney, two of which were apparently spent in detention, he seemed a changed man. Sure, he continued to do his job of meticulous hospital administration and record supervision, but somehow his enthusiasm for military protocol seemed to have petered out. Life as we knew it returned to normal.

Chapter Seventeen

True Colors

In the end, it turned out Parker wasn't such a bad guy after all. In fact, after the Sydney incident, he began hanging out with us quite a bit. To celebrate the good show of sportsmanship displayed by Parker and his lifer colleagues, and for other miscellaneous reasons, Hootch 8 threw yet another big party a few weeks later, complete with food, drink, and music. Roger Crumley played his guitar accompanied by the Filipino virtuosos, the guys sang along badly, and we welcomed several new arrivals.

Jehan Mir, a thoracic surgeon hailing from Pakistan, was a friendly and charming fellow who nevertheless we all felt sorry for. Despite the fact that he was not a U.S. citizen, he had somehow been drafted after his residency training and now here he was with us in Vietnam. Mir introduced us all to the traditions of Ramadan. I can still remember being awakened in the middle of the night by the sounds of cooking and the pungent smell of fried onions. During Ramadan, we soon learned, it was forbidden to eat or drink during daylight hours, and besides, Mir liked to prepare his own food. He also prayed five times a day, when work allowed, prostrating himself toward Mecca on his green prayer rug as we all watched in silence. A devout Muslim, he never drank alcohol in any form, sticking to Coke, orange juice, and tea.

Bob Rashti, another new arrival, was a neurosurgeon-in-training from Norfolk, whose small stature and black mustache reminded us all of Charlie Chaplin, especially since he continuously regaled us with his dry humor and colorful outfits – including a Charlie Chaplin-type derby hat. How had he found such a hat in Vietnam?

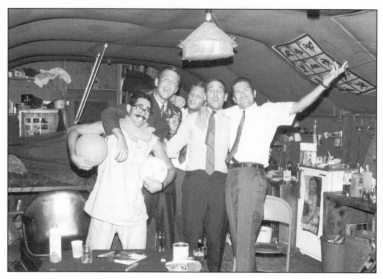

Hootch 8 party, L to R: Rashti, Whitney, Widmeyer, Crumley, Brief

So there we all were at the party, schmoozing, drinking, and eating, when suddenly, out of the blue, Rob Kaufmann stood up and began singing the opening words of the German anthem "*Deutschland, Deutschland über alles*" ("Germany, Germany above all") at the top of his lungs. Some guys seemed amused. I was not.

"Rob, please," I said, "not that, not here."

He wouldn't stop, and instead began singing louder.

"Please, Rob," I said, "you're in my hootch, you know how I feel about that stuff. Now I'm asking you nicely to stop. Please!"

To no avail. He then held his hand to his chest, his other hand hoisting a beer, as he bellowed again, "*Deutschland, Deutschland über alles...*"

I walked over to the bar, grabbed a pitcher of orange juice, and poured it over his head. He stopped singing, sputtered and coughed, then screamed: "Brief, you sonofabitch Jew bastard, I'll kill you! I swear, I'll frag your hootch!"

He lunged forward, swinging. I leaned back, but too late, getting clipped on the left cheek. I spun sideways and popped him a solid right to the gut. We grappled for a moment but were quickly restrained, Rob caught from behind in a bear hug by Gary Gregersen, while I was held back by Whitney and Crumley.

The party had come to a grinding halt as everybody stood around us, watching in silence. Then the Skipper walked over.

"Kaufmann, you made a serious threat against a fellow officer, I need to see you in my office at 0700."

He then walked out, casting a short wave to the rest of the group. Everyone dispersed back to their quarters. I sat on my bunk rubbing my cheek, feeling responsible for having sabotaged the party.

"Ahh, don't feel bad, Brief," said Crumley, slumping down in a chair next to me. "You're not the only one being called names. I've heard that prick Kaufmann make racist remarks about Alafriz too."

I shrugged.

"Yeah," continued Roger, "that's right. He's been known to make hints that he resents working under a 'gook' as head of anesthesia."

We all hit the sack, but despite all the beer, I kept going over the evening's events in my mind, wishing I had simply ignored Rob's singing.

The next morning, the Skipper gave Kaufmann a good dressing down, advising him that he was being written up, a letter of reprimand going into his permanent military record. The fact that the fragging threat had been made in a moment of passion fueled by alcohol, the Skipper informed him, was no excuse. His behavior was unbecoming of a naval officer, and if there was a recurrence, it would result in a court martial.

The reason I know what the Skipper said is because later that day, Kaufmann walked into Hootch 8, told me what had happened, and apologized.

"Apology accepted," I said, shaking his hand and thinking to myself that perhaps the punishment had exceeded the crime. Or maybe it hadn't.

Chapter Eighteen

Clinique Phuoc Thieu

Within weeks of my arrival at First Med, I realized that I needed a diversion from war, something to occupy my mind besides the constant crushing work, something to shield my sanity. I soon learned that I could volunteer my medical services. So on my days off, with the approval of the Skipper and the military authorities, I began working at a local civilian hospital in Danang.

On Wednesdays, at 0700, I would hitch a ride into town on the motor pool shuttle, returning to First Med by 2000. Clinique Phuoc Thieu, or CPT as the hospital was called, was housed in a large converted French colonial mansion with some eighty hospital beds, offering a wide range of medical services. I felt appreciated there, as I was the only orthopod at the hospital besides an elderly Vietnamese man who had been forced out of retirement. All the younger doctors had been conscripted into military hospitals.

I ran a clinic in the morning, treating sprains, fractures, and other ailments. In the afternoon, I worked in the OR, fixing severe fractures, dislocations, and other problems. The staff was extremely solicitous, treating me like royalty, and did all the preliminary prep work. I found it rewarding, even soothing, to work on patients who were not torn apart, not bleeding from every limb, patients whose surgery I could plan in a methodical fashion. This was exactly what I needed to maintain my mental stability and clinical judgment, not to mention my surgical skills.

The nursing staff was made up of nuns, mostly Vietnamese, but also a few British, French, and American volunteers. I encountered a major problem in my work at the hospital, and that was the lack of modern, up-to-date orthopedic equipment and supplies. Most of the time, I had to scramble and make do with outdated metallic hardware. But we managed, thanks to the competent nursing staff, as well as the patients themselves, who all seemed to have a remarkably high tolerance for pain.

Although most of my cases were routine surgeries, one stands out in my memory. About two months after I arrived in Nam, a sixty-five-year-old Vietnamese woman was brought in with a fractured femur, having been knocked down by a motor scooter while crossing the street. Her fracture, located just above the knee joint (supracondylar), was unstable and required ORIF with an L-shaped metallic blade-plate and screws. The problem was, the hospital had no such device. I therefore placed her in a hospital bed with leg traction, and as her circulation seemed intact, I planned to operate the following Wednesday.

While I was aware we were not allowed to take hardware from First Med for use on Vietnamese civilians, I also knew there was a large cabinet in the ortho clinic filled with old, damaged, discarded, or previously used hardware. After a thorough search, I found an ancient stainless steel L-shaped blade-plate with eight holes, bent but serviceable, which I thought would do the job.

I consulted with Mondello, our supply corpsman, who told me I was welcome to take the damaged device, since we had a full set of new blade-plates for use on wounded Marines. I then met with the Skipper, who also gave me his go-ahead. My next stop was the motor pool repair shop, where I hammered the plate into a useable state.

On the following Wednesday, I made an eight-inch lateral incision in the lower half of the thigh, exposing the entire distal half of the femur. I then used an osteotome to fashion a channel in the distal femur just above the knee joint and parallel to it. After that, I hammered the blade part of the device into the femur, driving it in until the plate touched the lateral femoral shaft.

At that point, I reduced the fracture fragments anatomically and held the whole thing together with a Lowman clamp. I then drove screws into all eight holes, catching both the medial and lateral cortex with each screw. The fracture solidly fixed, I closed up the incision.

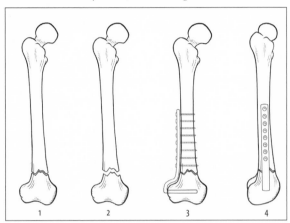

Femur fracture supracondylar
1. Supracondylar fracture of femur   2. Fracture is displaced
3. ORIF with 90 degree blade-plate and eight cortical screws   4. Side view showing plate and screw heads

Post-op x-rays showed that the fracture and hardware were in satisfactory position. Two days later, the patient began to walk with crutches and was discharged soon thereafter. I saw her in my clinic every couple weeks, and she was progressing well. Three months post-ORIF, she seemed nearly fully healed, and was able to walk comfortably with a cane.

Imagine my surprise when, six months later, another Vietnamese mamasan in her seventies came in with the same exact supracondylar femur fracture. This time I had no hardware to use on her, leaving me with a serious dilemma. Should I bring back woman A, then nine months post-op, remove her plate, and use it on woman B? I knew that in such fractures, hardware removal under one year from insertion ran the risk of re-fracture. But feeling I had no choice, I reluctantly decided to go ahead with it.

We brought woman A back to clinic, where x-rays showed full solid fracture healing. With her consent, I then proceeded to remove her blade-plate and screws, and after thorough cleaning and sterilizing, used them to fix woman B's fracture.

Both procedures went well, until the following week, when woman A was brought back in with a painful, swollen thigh: the femur had re-fractured along the original fracture line. I cursed myself for having taken the chance, for going against protocol, for showing poor judgment.

As the fracture was not displaced, I placed woman A in a thigh-high cast and put her back on crutches. Five weeks later, I rotated out of Nam, but I stayed in touch by mail with my orthopedic replacement at CPT. He advised me that some three months later she had healed well, and was again out of her cast, walking comfortably with a cane. He also reassured me that she did not seem angry and that every time she came to the clinic, she gave him a friendly black-toothed smile. Regardless, I was aware that back in the US, my decision would surely have resulted in a malpractice action. But then again, back in the US I would never have been faced with such a dilemma.

Several weeks after I began working at CPT, Sister Agatha, a British nun and OR nurse, arrived. Exceedingly well trained and knowledgeable in orthopedics, she would assist me in both the clinic and the OR, assuming a good share of the workload and facilitating my surgeries. As her lodging was on hospital grounds, she often invited a bunch of us back to her place after work, where we would sit and talk while Sister Aggie, as we called her, prepared drinks and dinner.

Our group consisted of the volunteer physicians and nurses, mostly Dutch, Italians, and Scandinavians. I was the only American. Our conversations tended to be animated, philosophical, and most entertaining.

Maurizio Chiappa, a vivacious and worldly OB/GYN from Florence, possessed a deep knowledge and appreciation of the fine arts, with particular fondness for the work of Botticelli, Tiepolo, Canaletto, and the other great Italian masters. His familiarity with just about every painting exhibited at the Uffizzi Galleries and the Pitti Palace in Florence was uncanny.

"Maurizio," I teased him one evening, "Is your great love of Botticelli explained by the superbly beautiful women he painted, or do you mostly appreciate his technique?"

"It's the women! I know this man!" quipped Piet Van der Meersch, a jovial surgeon from Amsterdam, as everyone laughed.

"The women, of course," admitted a smiling Maurizio. "No one has ever painted a female as exquisite as his *Birth of Venus* standing on that gigantic shell."

"Well, maybe Sorbi," I added.

"Who?" asked a puzzled Sister Aggie.

"Raffaello Sorbi," I continued. "Nineteenth century Florentine genre painter known for his extremely beautiful women. But I suppose the all-time champion of the idealized female beauty would probably be Ingres."

"Tell me, Paul," said a puzzled Maurizio, "how does an American orthopedic surgeon know about art?"

"I majored in fine arts at Columbia College," I answered. "And I grew up in Paris, where the museums are almost as nice as in Florence."

"Ah, Paris!" said Piet. "So you must be a lover of the Impressionists."

"Of course," I said. "Who doesn't love the Impressionists?"

"And which one of them is your favorite?" asked Maurizio. "Monet, Renoir, Degas, or Cezanne?"

"You know," I answered, "when I was younger, I loved all of them. Then my tastes changed, and Camille Pissarro became my favorite Impressionist. I love his beautiful scenes of crowded Paris boulevards and bridges, with strolling people and horse-drawn carriages. I have this fantasy that if I ever become very rich, I'll have a beautiful Pissarro hanging in my living room."

"Why did your tastes change?" asked Piet.

"It's complicated," I explained, "but mainly it has to do with two things: my being Jewish in France, and French anti-semitism."

"What?" exclaimed Maurizio. "You're Jewish? That's amazing! I am Jewish too!"

"You are?" I was shocked. "Maurizio Chiappa from Florence, a Jew?"

"Yes, we are Italian Jews for many generations, possibly all the way back to the Spanish Inquisition in 1492, when our ancestors were expelled from Gerona in Spain, and fled to Italy."

I was fascinated by Maurizio's revelation. But I was even more curious to know how he had survived World War II.

Maurizio explained that his family had hid in a monastery on the outskirts of Livorno, a port city on the western coast of Tuscany, where his mother was passed off as a nun, his father as a deacon, and little Maurizio was placed in the orphanage. He added that a number of their Jewish friends and relatives had been similarly sheltered by Catholic priests and nuns, who knowingly risked their lives to save Italian Jews from deportation to death camps. The room fell silent and I sensed that Sister Aggie felt proud.

"Paul," said Maurizio, breaking the silence, "tell us about the French anti-semitism, I am curious."

"Well, besides a basic undercurrent of anti-semitism found in most European countries, France had the peculiar problem of the Dreyfus Affair. Any of you know about the Dreyfus Affair?"

They did not. I explained that in 1894, Alfred Dreyfus, a French army captain and a Jew, was falsely accused of spying for Germany. After being found guilty in a highly publicized military trial, he was publicly humiliated, stripped of his rank, and sentenced to life imprisonment on Devil's Island, a tropical disease-infested hellhole off the coast of South America.

The Dreyfus case generated a tidal wave of vicious anti-semitism among the French, who were still aching from their humiliating defeat in the Franco-Prussian War of 1870–1871. Anti-Jewish sentiment flared all over France, with massive street riots, pogrom-style beatings of Jews, as well as the stoning and burning of Jewish homes and businesses. France became bitterly divided between Dreyfus-haters and those who believed him innocent.

In 1898, Emile Zola, the famed French novelist, published a full front-page letter titled "I accuse," in a prominent Paris newspaper, in which he openly accused the French government and the French army of fraud, claiming that Captain Dreyfus had been framed and wrongly convicted on trumped-up charges of espionage.

The case was blown wide open. Dreyfus was brought back from Devil's Island, retried, exonerated, and eventually fully restored into the French army with the rank of major. But the damage had already been done. Despite Dreyfus's exoneration, millions of French remained bitterly anti-semitic.

"So how did that affect your taste in art?" Maurizio finally asked.

"Well," I answered, "it turns out Degas and Cezanne were fierce Jew haters. That tainted my personal appreciation of their work, something I am not particularly proud of. On the other hand, Pissarro, who was himself a Jew, understandably sided with Dreyfus and that influenced me as well. But over and above all that, I just love the way Pissarro painted."

We talked about France and art for a while longer.

"But don't forget, my friends," said Piet Van der Meersch with obvious pride, "don't forget Vincent Van Gogh in all this, perhaps the greatest, most sublime painter of all time…and a Dutchman like me!"

We all laughed. I agreed in a way. Van Gogh unquestionably stood alone, unique in his style, his colors, his compositions, and his great mystique.

We talked back and forth like that for hours, moving on to discussing modern greats like Picasso, Magritte, and my favorite American painter, Edward Hopper. I felt as if I were in art heaven, along with some very art-savvy friends.

But invariably, at some point in the evening, we would end up discussing the Vietnam war. As the only US serviceman in the room, I often found myself on the defensive.

"Face it, Paul, this war is pointless," said Piet. "And your soldiers are dying for nothing. The US shouldn't even be here. What's the point?"

"The point is communism," I replied.

"Communism? That's all? Please explain."

"Okay, if you want my humble opinion, I'll give you my take on why we're here. You have this Asian country, northern half communist, southern half not. North tries to conquer south, so the US comes in on the southern side with troops, equipment, support, and now you've got a war. What country am I talking about?"

"Vietnam, of course!" exclaimed Maurizio.

"No, it was a trick question. I was actually talking about Korea."

"Korea? So what's your point?" asked Piet.

"My point is simply that our reasons for getting involved in Korea and Vietnam were very similar, namely to stem the tide of communism."

"Do you mean to tell us that Korea and Vietnam are the same?" asked Piet.

"No, not the wars, just the basic reason for getting involved, which again, is communism."

"So what are the differences?" asked Maurizio.

"I guess the principal difference is that in Korea we won, whereas in Vietnam victory seems elusive."

"Why is it elusive? Aren't you much stronger and better equipped than North Vietnam?"

"We are," I conceded, "but there are factors working against us in Vietnam which give the enemy some distinct advantages."

"What factors?" asked Sister Agatha.

"A number of them. I hope I'm not boring you, so please bear with me on this. First, in Korea, we had on our side a true military genius called General Douglas MacArthur. Some people think he turned the tide of the war in our favor through sheer military brilliance. In Vietnam, no such luck, as the military genius seems to be on the enemy's side, namely General Giap."

"Giap?" queried Maurizio. "Who is Giap?"

"Vo Nguyen Giap," I continued, "the brilliant, tenacious pit bull of a man who in 1954 defeated the French at Dien Bien Phu, and is now supreme commander of all communist forces in Vietnam, answering only to Ho Chi Minh. We have no such brilliant generals on our side today. Our top brass is good, but not great.

"Second, the people back in the US hate this war. There are weekly war protests, people burning draft cards. With Korea, while people were not enthusiastic in their support, at least there were no mass rallies, no anti-war marches on Washington. Nobody seemed to hate the war then.

"Third, Korea was not a guerilla war. The engagements, difficult and murderous as they were, were mostly strategic battles between uniformed troops. In Nam, the Vietcong guerilla fighters are unrecognizable. They wear no uniforms, they mix with the population, and work mainly at night. How do you fight an enemy you cannot see or recognize?

"Fourth, is the Vietnamese people themselves. In South Korea, the people were truly united in wanting to hold off communism, truly interested in fighting for their freedom, while here in South Vietnam, the people seem confused, disinterested, resigned to whatever happens.

"Fifth and possibly most important, is that we are being forced to fight with one hand tied behind our back. The troops feel that the US is not fighting this war to win it. In 1945, Truman ended the war in the Pacific by dropping two atom bombs on Japan. Mind you, I'm not suggesting we should nuke North Vietnam, but I cannot understand why we don't at least bomb Hanoi, or consider invading the north. We just don't seem fully committed to winning this war."

I apologized for being long-winded, but added that I had a bad feeling about what would happen once the Americans eventually pulled out.

"You seem kind of resigned to losing this war yourself," said Maurizio. "What do you think will be the outcome?"

"I really don't know," I said. "Some sort of negotiated peace, I suppose. But hey, I'm a doctor, not a politician. What do I know about this stuff?"

We all sat in silence for a while.

Similar discussions took place every week, so that I eventually began to feel like I belonged to a French "salon" in the eighteenth century, where intellectual discussions flourished. And I suppose my explanation of our involvement in Vietnam had its effect, because after that discussion, I definitely felt less on the defensive. In the late evening, I would catch the last shuttle vehicle back to First Med and the weekly routine became a pleasant diversion, a welcome relief from the stresses of war.

After several months, I noticed that our discussion group was getting noticeably smaller, and one afternoon I arrived at Sister Agatha's apartment after surgery to find myself alone with her. Thinking nothing of it, I discussed the day's surgeries, and after dinner, I left. The following week, and the week after that, it was again just the two of us. And I liked it. We sat closer and closer on her couch, as it became apparent to both of us that our friendship was beginning to transcend the platonic.

Our relationship lasted for months, until the end of my Vietnam tour, and remained a closely guarded secret. I never spoke of it to my colleagues at First Med and to my knowledge, no one at CPT ever became aware of it. If either of us harbored any guilt, she for breaking her vows and I for facilitating her transgression, we never openly discussed it. It was a time of great turmoil and greater loneliness, and both of us held on to what we had for as long as we could. We asked each other no painful questions, for fear of bursting what seemed to be a most fragile bubble.

While my association with Sister Agatha at the hospital remained professional, what transpired afterhours assumed a surreal, dreamlike quality. Though we both knew our relationship was bound to become yet another victim of the war, we seldom spoke of that, preferring to simply live the short time we had together. The fatalistic realism we both harbored made the unavoidable easier to bear, and when the time came for us to part, no tears were shed. Almost.

Chapter Nineteen

Passover 1970

On April 15, 1970, I was approached by Father Vincennes, our Catholic chaplain.

"Dr. Brief, you're Jewish, correct?"

"Yes I am, Father, why do you ask?"

"Did you know that next week is Passover?"

I shook my head. Not only was I unaware that Passover was approaching, I realized that I had completely missed the High Holy Days of Rosh Hashanah and Yom Kippur the previous September. I vaguely remembered my mother mentioning the holidays in a September letter soon after my arrival in Nam. But with the carnage, the stress, and the sleepless nights, these holidays had passed right by me.

"No, Father," I said with a touch of guilt. "I had no notion. I guess this place doesn't much lend itself to religious observance, as I'm sure you know."

"Only too well," he sighed. "But I've received notice that they're holding a Passover Seder next week at the Air Force base in Danang, and all Jewish personnel are invited. I'll send you a notice with all the details."

"Thank you, Father."

I mentioned this to the Skipper and after getting his approval, made arrangements for a ride with the motor pool.

At 1700 on April 20, three of us, including myself, our dentist Lt. Marc Blumberg, and a Jewish Marine sergeant named Bielski, all dressed in clean jungle fatigues, boots shined and caps starched, boarded a shuttle bus and rode one hour to the I-Corps Air Force base north of Danang. As instructed, we walked up to a large hangar and after entering the open doors, came upon a remarkable sight.

The entire hangar, approximately the size of a football field, was filled with long tables arranged in neat rows, at which sat a sea of men wearing white yarmulkes. We were handed ours by a chaplain standing at the door, then were pointed in the direction of a table with available seating. I stood at my seat for a moment just looking around, awed by the sheer spectacle of a multitude of men in green uniforms with little white caps, the whole tableau reminiscent of a gigantic green meadow strewn with white flowers. There were maybe two thousand of us there that evening. I wondered if this many Jewish American soldiers had ever been assembled together before.

We sat and chatted, exchanging names and shaking hands. The men hailed from all over the map: Chicago, Boston, Dallas, even an Army major from Anchorage, Alaska.

"What's the Jewish population of Anchorage?" I asked.

"You're looking at it!" he answered to a round of laughter. "What's the Jewish population of New York?"

"Not much," I replied, pointing to the crowded hall, "looks like we're all here!" More laughter.

Then a tall, distinguished-looking older man in jungle fatigues walked up to the raised podium and spoke into the microphone.

"Gentlemen, I am Rabbi Eliezer Grossman, Jewish chaplain for I-Corps. I welcome you all to our Passover Seder for the year 5730" – long round of applause and cheers – "... and I'd like to begin our service with this invocation. Please rise."

We all stood, with eyes on the rabbi, who spoke in a solemn voice:

"Almighty God, we thank you for allowing so many of us to gather here to celebrate Passover. Although we are each and every one of us

thousands of miles away from our families back home, we are grateful for being together here today as a family of soldiers. Please God, safeguard these Jewish servicemen, together with all their gentile comrades, shield them from harm, and allow them all to return home in safety and in good health, so that next year they may celebrate Passover together with their loved ones in America. Just as you shielded your Jewish flock during the exodus from Egypt by thwarting Pharaoh's efforts to destroy us, so shield these men gathered here today and keep them safe from harm. Please allow them to serve their country with distinction, then grant them a safe passage home so they may be returned to their waiting families in good health, in good spirits, in peace and intact.

O Lord, in these most dangerous of times, we humbly ask for your divine protection and we thank you for your benevolence, for your loving kindness, and for this Passover Seder.

And let us say: Amen."

The entire crowd intoned a loud Amen in unison, and as I looked around, I saw there was not a dry eye in the room. The rabbi, assisted by his fellow Jewish chaplains, then proceeded to conduct a full Passover Seder, complete with the Four Questions, the matzohs, the bitter herbs, the charoset, and the listing of the Ten Plagues inflicted on Pharaoh and his people. The meal, served to us by Air Force volunteers, had all the traditional Seder foods: gefilte fish with horseradish, chicken soup with matzoh balls, roasted chicken with potatoes, followed by fruit and honey cake. There was even kosher wine. It was the closest thing to being home I'd experienced in nine months.

I was feeling emotional as I realized what a huge effort it must have been to organize such an event. I thought to myself that someday, when I have children, I will tell them about Passover in Vietnam in 1970, an event which, to this day, symbolizes for me America's good faith and tolerance. I felt proud to be a Jewish military officer in the service of my country, grateful to realize that the respect I had for America was mutual.

That evening, riding back to First Med in the shuttle vehicle, I thought back to the fleeting idea I'd once entertained of running off to

Canada, and realized it would have been the mistake of my life. It felt right for me to be in Vietnam. I felt I belonged here.

As we walked back to our respective hootches, I waved goodnight to Blumberg. Little did I suspect he would not be with us much longer.

Chapter Twenty

Dr. Blumberg

Marc Joshua Blumberg, our battalion dentist, considered himself more of a Marine than a dentist. Though a reservist like most of us, with no military career aspirations, he demonstrated an uncanny affinity for all things military, and was often seen walking around in pressed and starched jungle fatigues, toting his M16 rifle, his .45 on his hip, plus a 357 Magnum in a shoulder holster. The guy had a definite John Wayne complex, and we used to joke that it actually made sense for our dentist to be "armed to the teeth."

While the rest of us went to mandatory target practice every few weeks, Blumberg practiced regularly, gleefully firing his assorted arsenal for hours on end. That was harmless enough; what concerned us was that he had actually convinced Captain Larkin, the CO of our Marine garrison, to let him go up on Huey helicopter gunships for nighttime combat missions. The next day, he'd gush about how thrilling it was to see the long streaks of tracer bullets at night, how Captain Larkin had let him fire the M60 machine guns at Charlie, and how exciting it was to watch the bandoliers of M60 rounds dancing into the gun from the left side while the shells popped out on the right. In short, the man was a nut. And he kept going up on those Hueys again and again.

About a week after Passover, Blumberg was apparently taking part in a night action when his chopper came under heavy ground fire. He must have been leaning forward because an AK47 round shot right through the chopper floor and struck him just behind the chin, lodging in his tongue. Knocked unconscious by the impact, Blumberg was immediately medevaced back to First Med, where he regained consciousness. However, he had such massive lingual swelling that he couldn't speak, and could breathe only through his nose.

After skull x-rays were taken, Crumley, our ENT expert, took him right to the OR. Alafriz had to perform a nasotracheal intubation, inserting the anesthesia tube through the nose, past the pharynx into the trachea, instead of the usual way through the back of the mouth.

While he was in the OR, I ran over to triage and looked at the x-rays. It was astonishing, the most shocking film I'd seen since the one showing the femur near the heart. There was the entire skull with a huge AK47 round sitting upright like Stonehenge, right between his upper and lower teeth where the tongue normally sits. Blumberg was lucky that the bullet had first shot through the helicopter fuselage, spending most of its energy, otherwise the round would have shot right through the top of his head and killed him. The man was as lucky as he was mad, or had Rabbi Grossman's Passover prayer saved his life?

I walked back to Hootch 8 and about a half hour later heard the squawkbox: "Dr. Brief to OR, Dr. Brief to OR STAT!"

As I rushhed into OR 2, Crumley explained the situation:

"I went in, retracted his mouth open with dental padding, then located and removed the bullet easily enough with an incision under the tongue. Usual lingual bleeding, nothing out of the ordinary. But when I got through suturing up my sublingual incision and tried to close his mouth, I could not. Seems we must have pried his mouth open too wide, and dislocated his jaw. You have experience with that?"

"Absolutely," I reassured him. "I trained at HJD in New York City, where the ER is super busy with all kinds of trauma including Saturday Night Specials like broken and dislocated jaws, so I had my share of those. But first, let's get a lateral x-ray of his head to confirm the dislocation."

While waiting for the portable x-ray, I quickly put on gloves and checked the patient. Sure enough, the jaw was dislocated, both TMJs having popped out of place with the mandibular condyles slipped forward where I could actually feel them with my gloved thumbs. The x-ray tech arrived with the portable machine and shot a quick lateral skull x-ray, which confirmed the dislocation.

I turned to Alafriz:

"Sonny, please give me the maximum muscle relaxation possible so I can pop this thing back into place."

I heavily padded my thumbs with gauze, as dislocated jaws can snap back into place quite violently and bite your hand. Then I pressed down and backwards with my thumbs on both sides of the mandible inside the mouth, while pivoting the back of the jaw forward with my fingers from outside the face. A loud clunk followed and the jaw snapped shut on my thumbs, which thankfully were padded enough to prevent injury. Crumley then pried the jaw open just enough to allow my thumbs to escape.

"Thanks Rog, I needed that!"

"Brief, nice work, I owe you one!"

"You owe me nothing, pal. Well…maybe just a nice chorus of 'Proud Mary' later with your guitar and a couple of beers."

I walked out, leaving Crumley and Alafriz chuckling. The next day I was sitting at Blumberg's bedside. Unable to eat or speak because of a massively swollen tongue, he was being fed intravenously, and also drank liquids through a specially designed straw Crumley had fabricated out of a piece of quarter-inch copper pipe borrowed from the Seabees. As I sat there talking to him, he responded by writing on a legal pad.

"Blumberg, you are one lucky dentist! Talk is you're getting a Purple Heart, and you're going home."

"I'd rather stay here," he wrote.

"Yeah, yeah," I replied. "I'd like to be in your place, going home and all. And besides, everybody thinks I talk too much anyway."

He smiled and wrote: "Crumley told me what happened. Thanks for relocating my jaw!"

"My pleasure, and thank *you* for not biting my thumbs off. But do you realize how lucky you were? If that AK round hadn't spent most of its energy piercing the chopper floor before it hit you, it would've probably blown your brains out!"

He smiled and nodded in agreement.

"Not that you dentist types have that much brains to blow out…"

He laughed and wrote: "Please don't make me laugh, it hurts my tongue."

"Say, Blumberg," I continued, "are you aware you're probably the only dentist in US military history to get a Purple Heart?"

He nodded and wrote "I doubt it."

"Okay, let me rephrase that: you're probably the only *Jewish* dentist in US military history…"

With that he agreed and mouthed "maybe."

"Anyhow, just to get serious for a moment," I continued, "when you get back home to Philadelphia, you should go to your local synagogue and say the *Bentsch Gomel* prayer."

He scribbled, "What's that?"

"*Oy vey,* Blumberg, seems you're even less Jewish than I am. It's a prayer of thanks recited before the Torah after you've had a close call, or a brush with death. And you, my friend, have certainly had a brush with death…"

We shook hands, he mouthed "thanks again," and I left. Two days later, our fearless warrior dentist left for home. Lucky man indeed, with a great story to tell his grandchildren.

Chapter Twenty-One

Donald Duffy

Sometime after I returned from Vietnam, it occurred to me that of the thousands of GIs I treated, I could not remember a single soldier's name. Not a single one – except for Donald Duffy. Donald Duffy's case was so sad, so heartbreakingly tragic, that he came to symbolize the entire war to me.

On May 13, I was called to triage to see yet another double amputee. As I walked over, I envisioned the by-now familiar scene: a young GI with both legs blown off, stumps bleeding and black with soot and dirt and burning flesh, emitting a steady, low groan of pain and despair. I was still sickened and distressed by each and every case, but having been through it so many times since that initial case back in August 1969 when I had my first encounter with water buffalo feces, I had become somewhat hardened to it by dint of sheer repetition.

Yet the Donald Duffy nightmare exceeded anything I'd seen before. There he lay, with both legs blown off at mid-thigh, steaming with burning flesh and hanging tendons and muscles. But that wasn't even half the horror of it. In place of his genitals was a huge, gaping hole reaching into his pelvis. His right arm was missing, amputated above the elbow. With a flail chest, he already had two chest tubes connected to suction devices. His face was heavily bandaged and a tracheostomy tube emerged from his bandaged neck.

I learned from the corpsman in the medevac chopper that when Donald tripped the unusually powerful Bouncing Betty booby trap, he had been crouching forward and looking down. Consequently, he caught multiple shrapnel fragments in his chest and face in addition to his limbs. He was blinded, both orbits blown out.

While in the chopper, he went into respiratory arrest, but because of all the bleeding over his face and mouth, he could not be intubated. The corpsman decided to perform a tracheostomy right then and there to save his life. Because of the poor lighting and all the shaking, the tracheostomy became a difficult and brutal undertaking. Using a scalpel in the dark with a flashlight held by a Marine, and operating on a screaming soldier without anesthesia, the heroic corpsman experienced great difficulty in finding and opening the trachea. He managed to save the soldier's life, but in the process, he also mangled his vocal chords.

So there I was, looking at Donald Duffy, a twenty-year-old Marine who had lost both legs, his right arm, his genitals, his eyes, and his voice. He couldn't see, he couldn't speak, he couldn't move. But he could hear.

"Donald," I said into his right ear, "can you hear me?"

He nodded affirmatively.

"Donald, I'm Dr. Brief. You're safe now in an American hospital. I'm going to take care of you, and I have a whole bunch of doctor friends who are going to help me take care of you. You're going to be okay, and when you get better you'll be sent back home to the world, to your family. Do you understand me?"

He nodded yes.

I sent out for two more ortho teams, plus urology, thoracic, and ophthalmology. This was going to be a massive and grueling multispecialty effort.

We spent the entire day and most of the night cleaning and trimming his wounds. Widmeyer, Whitney, Kilroy, and Gregersen joined us in tending to his three amputated limbs. Roger Crumley and Sterling Trenberth, the opthalmologist, teamed up in addressing his tracheostomy, his face, and his eyes. Thoracic surgeon Jehan Mir replaced his chest tubes, monitored his breathing, and controlled the suction devices to keep his lungs inflated. Meanwhile, Alafriz kept him under anesthesia, careful to utilize a minimum of gas, monitoring his blood volume, and transfusing him a total of thirty-two units of blood during the many hours of surgery he required.

Urologist Bill Bauer managed to pass a specialized Foley tube into his bladder, somehow securing it directly to his pelvic wall with well-placed sutures. Trenberth evaluated and re-evaluated his eyes, then sadly informed us that his vision was irretrievably lost.

Every couple hours, the Skipper would step into the OR to see how things were going, and ask if we needed any additional help.

After some thirty-eight hours of continuous surgery by the various specialists, Lance Corporal Donald Duffy appeared to have stabilized. Sedated on a respirator, he was no longer bleeding from his wounds, his vital signs were stable, and he was putting out urine. Three days later, we took him off his respirator and to our great relief, he was able to breathe on his own.

And there he was. He couldn't move, he couldn't see, he couldn't speak. But he could hear, and he could write. So I would sit with him and ask him questions, and with a pencil I placed in his left hand, he would scribble answers on the pad which I held for him.

"Donald, where are you from?"

"Kimberly, Idaho," he wrote. "Not far from Twin Falls. My family runs a potato farm there."

"Oh, so now I'll think about you every time I eat a baked potato."

He smiled and wrote: "What's your name, Doc? Where you from?"

"I'm Dr. Brief, one of the doctors taking care of you. I'm from New York City."

"New York City," he wrote, "big scary place. Always wanted to go there."

"Someday you will, and you'll come visit me. And I'll take you to my favorite baked potato restaurant."

"Doc, why is it you're the only one comes talk to me?"

"I guess I've become attached to you, maybe because I was there the day you came in and I was the first doctor to work on you. But many doctors have worked on you, and together we saved your life."

"Why save my life?" he scribbled.

I was crying.

"Many reasons. Because your life is important. Because your family loves you. Also because you're a Marine, you're one of us. We love Marines here, and it's our job to save them. Do you have brothers and sisters?"

"Yes," he wrote, "three sisters and four brothers, and I'm the youngest. Dad and two brothers were Marines before me."

"When you get home, the whole family will care for you."

"Why should they care for me?"

"Because you're their son and their brother, and because you'll always be the Duffy family war hero."

"Doc, what about my legs? Can I ever walk again?"

"Absolutely. They'll fit your with prostheses and you'll be able to walk around just fine. They'll also fit you with a prosthetic arm and you'll be able to function like normal."

"What about my eyes? They hurt. Will I see again?"

"Too soon to tell," I lied. "The eye experts back home will work on you and you'll be amazed what those guys can do."

We conversed back and forth like that for at least an hour every day. I'd sneak out between OR cases, and tell him about the war and my life. Sometimes we just sat quietly and I held his hand.

"Donald, what happened to you? Were you walking point?"

"Don't remember. Just remember lots of pain, pain in my eyes."

Obviously his amnesia extended back a while, as I found out he'd been in-country only three months.

"What's the last thing you remember?"

"Remember boot camp. Pendleton."

"Hey, Pendleton! That's my boot camp! Pretty tough, right? Who was your drill instructor?"

"Gunny McAvoy," he scribbled, "toughest motherf…on earth."

"Boy, you got that right! McAvoy, I don't believe it! Donald, you and I, we seem to have a lot in common. We were even tortured by the same mean bastard!"

He smiled and nodded in agreement.

After some three weeks, when he no longer needed blood transfusions (he required a total of seventy units during his stay at First Med), and the medical team began talking of transferring him out to Japan, I went to see Captain Lea.

"Skipper," I said, "if it's at all possible, I'd like to request permission to fly escort on Duffy's medevac to Yokosuka. I wouldn't ask for this ordinarily, but being that it's him, I'd like to personally see to it that he has a safe flight."

"Well, Brief," he replied, "it's been a while since you've had a break, and I know you've grown quite attached to that heroic kid. I'll see what I can do."

And so on June 5, I went out on Donald Duffy's c-130 medevac flight. This time, no drama, no pulled-out chest tubes to replace. I sat by his side through the entire flight, talking to him and holding his hand, dozing off when he slept. He appeared calm and comfortable, with no complaints. I was awed by his strength and his courage.

When we arrived in Yokosuka, I personally discussed Donald with the RMO (receiving medical officer), giving him a quick synopsis of the case. I then went over to Donald, shook his hand, and told him I would contact him when I got home in a few months, making a real effort to keep my voice from cracking. He squeezed my hand hard and shook his head in appreciation, mouthing the words, "thank you for everything." I then wrote down the serial number on his dog tags for later reference, wiped my eyes, and walked out into the cool evening air to catch the train to Tokyo.

Chapter Twenty-Two

Tokyo Revisited

Tokyo felt different the second time around, somehow quieter, more sedate. Solange Lejeune-Ito was nowhere to be found. She was not at the Sanno, and her telephone number rang and rang with no answer. Perhaps the colonel had been reassigned. I wasn't really surprised; when we parted I'd had a strong intuition I would never see her again.

Her absence made me sad. Still, I felt an obligation to utilize my week in Tokyo to shake off my doldrums, aware that I could not go back to First Med in this condition. My hootchmates, my colleagues, my patients all deserved better, and I was going to find a way to cheer myself up. After a couple days of leisurely visits to the city's beautiful parks and stores, followed by evenings of drinking at the Sanno Hotel bar trading war stories with fellow Americans, I decided what the hell, I'd give the Yokohama Lounge another try.

And lo and behold, this time Yoko (aka Annie) was there, she was free, and she remembered Kilroy. Not only was she beautiful, she was everything Killjoy had said she was, and more. A sort of geisha, she was extremely charming, friendly, vivacious, and knowledgeable. She took me to her apartment, which was surprisingly luxurious, where she cooked and sang and danced to Japanese music.

After a couple of days and nights with her, I clearly understood Killjoy's fascination with this woman. On our third day, she drove us to Maebashi, her hometown some fifty miles northwest of Tokyo, a quaint, peaceful place she knew inside and out. Like an expert tour guide, she took me to two museums, art galleries, a Shinto temple, some gorgeous waterfalls, and a lake with magnificent black swans. At my insistence, we ate lunch and dinner several times at the same excellent restaurant, with the most fastidious service one could imagine. She had wanted to take me to another restaurant for dinner, but after that first lunch, I longed to repeat the magic. I was not disappointed. I had never tried hot sake before, but it sure went well with the steamed squid and shiitake mushrooms in black bean sauce. This was followed by a superb plum wine that complemented our tender Kobe beef. I never dreamt I could experience such hedonistic delights in a small Japanese town, right in the middle of all the Vietnam misery.

After three days together, my mood had taken a definite turn for the better. The following evening, back in Tokyo, Yoko took me to a Kabuki theater. Although I understood not a single word, I found the spectacle fascinating, especially the intricate mask-like makeup and elaborate costumes. Close to midnight, we ate a late supper at a popular sushi restaurant in the Ginza. In 1970, sushi had yet to gain a foothold in the US, which meant I had never eaten raw fish before. Weird but enjoyable, I liked the soy sauce mixed with wasabi, a strange green paste that tasted like a combination of horseradish and mustard. Patiently and expertly, Yoko taught me the art of using chopsticks.

My time with Yoko was a five-day crash course in all things Japanese, a course which covered culture, music, geography, and culinary arts. We even went to a Sumo wrestling match, which I found astonishing not for the sport, but for the sheer monstrous size of these creatures, most of whom weighed between four hundred and six hundred pounds, dwarfing our comically pumped-up professional wrestlers back home.

When it came time to leave, I soon understood how Yoko could afford her lifestyle, including her apartment, her car, and her beautiful clothes. She actually never mentioned money, and when I asked what I owed her, she acted coy and sheepish. I knew what I had to do, so I simply gave her all the money I'd brought with me, thinking she deserved even more. She thanked me, bowed deeply, then drove me to Yokosuka. After a sad goodbye, I boarded my plane for the return trip to Danang.

Back at First Med, Killjoy was envious that I had gotten together with Yoko "again," and amused to hear that her many attributes were every bit as remarkable as he had described them. My doldrums gone, I felt I was now ready to get back to work. But the truth was I hadn't been able to get Donald Duffy out of my mind, and I wondered how he was getting on.

Chapter Twenty-Three
Brig Attack

One week after my return from Tokyo, the principal Marine Corps brig in 1-Corps was blown up by the Vietcong. Starting at 0300 on May 19, heavy casualties began pouring in by the truckload and chopperload as the entire medical staff was summoned to triage. By 0800, we had received some 283 casualties, half of them severe. There were multiple massive injuries – fractured limbs, skulls, faces, and spines. Many were open injuries caused by shrapnel, while others were crush injuries resulting from caved-in prison walls. Some of the injuries had been caused by high falls due to collapsed floors.

This was a mass casualty in the truest sense, and our staff's triage skills were put to the test. Under the expert guidance of our chief triage officer Dr. Sam Winner, we quickly grouped the wounded according to the severity and life-threatening gradient of their injuries. Most severe was group one, unconscious personnel with penetrating injuries to the head and face. Then came group two, with chest injuries that threatened the heart and lungs. Group three was composed of soldiers suffering from penetrating abdominal wounds, which caused massive internal bleeding. Group four covered severe limb injuries, mostly open fractures with or without vascular compromise. Group five was comprised of guys with closed fractures and missile injuries, which appeared to pose no threat to life or limb.

Most of the men in the first three groups needed to be taken to the OR STAT, and each of our six ORs was triply set up to accommodate the volume. We all assisted one another and I found myself working in thoracic, urology, and general surgery, while our colleagues in turn assisted us with multiply fractured patients. Working at high speed, we must have looked like characters in the old silent movies. All surgeons and corpsmen worked non-stop for nearly seventy-two hours, with only short breaks to catch a hurried meal or change our blood-soaked scrubs.

At about 2200 on the third day, First Med came under heavy attack by several VC platoons. They approached from the road bordering the hospital as well as from the back of the compound, where some had apparently scaled the ravine and engaged our Marine garrison in hand-to-hand combat. The scene was chaotic, with the earsplitting blasts of the plastique charges and the incessant rattle of small-arms fire. Meanwhile, helicopter gunships flew overhead spraying the area, streaking long rows of red tracers everywhere, careful to spare our personnel from friendly fire.

The air was filled with smoke and the smell of gunpowder. Even in the ORs we wore helmets and flak jackets under our scrub gowns, weapons strapped to our sides. I was working on a grunt with an open femur fracture when the OR door flew open and two men came running in. In a split-second of confusion, I dropped to one knee, tore my gown open, and reached for my .45, thinking that the enemy had burst into the OR. But the two intruders turned out to be Marines, who soon started yelling, "Incoming, incoming, hit the deck!!!"

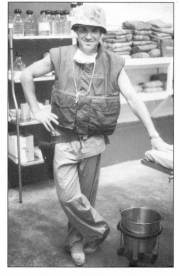

OR garb during enemy attacks

We all dove to the floor, the *ack-ack-ack-ack* of automatic weapons right on us. One second later, the wall on the right side of the OR blew open with a huge, deafening blast. We'd been hit by sappers, and for a moment I could hear nothing, temporarily deafened by the explosion. Smoke and dust were everywhere. Still lying on the OR floor, I saw the two Marines rush to the breached wall, where they quickly set up their M60 and began firing heavy volleys *tat-tat-tat-tat-tat-tat* at the enemy outside. Then I turned my head and from under my helmet saw a remarkable sight: Alafriz, lying on his back, was rhythmically squeezing the airbag to ventilate the patient's lungs, as the patient lay on the table under anesthesia. Sonny Alafriz – always on the job no matter what.

Finally, the attack appeared to be over. We stood up, and with Mondello's help, I quickly hung a hospital sheet to cover the breached wall. Mondello hosed down the patient's wounds, which had been covered with dust. Then we quickly scrubbed up, regowned, and resumed operating on the patient's femur. No big deal really, all in a day's work.

Later that night, after being relieved by Whitney to catch some sleep, I woke up in a sweat, shaking. I couldn't stop thinking about how I had almost opened fire on the two Marines, mistaking them for VC. Had it all been a nightmare, or did the OR wall really blow? I wasn't sure.

The following morning as I walked past the OR, I observed a group of Seabees rebuilding the damaged wall, happily hammering away as a boom box pounded out rock music. I stopped for a moment and smiled, remembering how much I'd always admired construction work back home. I thought, not for the first time, that in my next life I would like to be a carpenter – a real carpenter, not just an orthopedic one. As I stood there in my scrubs, one Seabee stopped hammering and yelled out, "It's no biggie, doc! We'll have this place all fixed up for ya *bookoo* quick!"

Chapter Twenty-Four

A Souvenir

It took First Med a full two weeks to treat and stabilize all the casualties from the brig explosion, and to repair the damage caused by the vc attack. Meanwhile, our normal daily load of combat injuries kept rolling in, and I found myself working frequently alongside Jim Lockhart.

Jim Lockhart was a skillful general surgeon from Tulsa who excelled in vascular surgery. When we worked together on complex, multiply injured limbs, he would address the soft tissue problems while I handled the fractures. One day, when a grunt caught an ak47 round in the thigh, resulting in a mid-shaft femur fracture and a severed femoral artery, we were both called to triage. In a two-minute conference held while viewing the x-rays, we mapped out a surgical plan.

"So, Paul," he said, "I'll start out, make an anterior thigh incision, then find and clamp off the two ends of the femoral artery. Then you take over, right?"

"Absolutely. You'll temporarily close your incision with a few sutures, then I'll turn the patient on his side and fix the femur. Because the x-ray shows a midshaft fracture with two main fragments and a large butterfly, I figure the best fixation would be a Kuntscher medullary nail with cerclage wires. Fast and stable, followed by a quick skin closure."

"Right," he continued, "then we turn him back supine, I harvest my saphenous vein for the interposition graft, measure off the proper length, then reverse the graft and suture it to both ends of the artery. Done. Okay?"

We agreed and went off to the OR, where Alafriz already had the patient asleep, and corpsman Radcliffe had prepared a full double setup for both vascular and ortho. The plan was right out of the FSMS manual, which had indoctrinated us that in cases of limb injury combining fractures and vascular damage, it was imperative to first obtain bone stability before attempting vascular repair. The reason was that if the vascular work was done first, the fragile repair would be endangered by all the manipulating, bending, and hammering required for fracture fixation.

Our plan worked. Within an hour, I had the fracture solidly fixed with a Kuntscher nail that I had pre-measured using the normal thigh as a guide. To hold the butterfly fragment in place, I tightly secured two cerclage wires. This achieved a solid, stable fixation which could withstand limb movement, thus allowing the vascular repair graft to sit in a safe and secure environment.

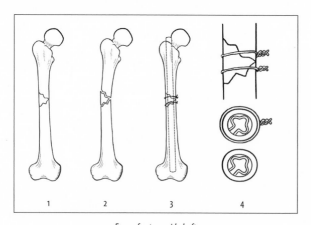

Femur fracture mid-shaft

1. Mid-shaft fracture of femur   2. Fracture is displaced, note butterfly fragment
3. ORIF with Kuntscher Nail and two cerclage wires   4. Top: close-up of butterfly fragment and cerclage wires

We then turned the patient on his back and Lockhart wasted no time as he quickly harvested his saphenous vein, flipped it, and did his grafting procedure in short order. X-rays showed good, solid fixation of the fracture, and the grunt's pedal pulses were bounding.

We decided to give the retrieved AK 47 round to the patient as a souvenir, and the next day, when I went to check on him, he was sitting up in bed, grinning and proudly displaying his trophy bullet, which hung from his dog tag chain. A buddy of his in the motor pool had apparently drilled a hole right through it.

Lockhart and I worked together on a number of cases, but one in particular stands out in my memory. Late in June, as many of us were turning into "short-timers," Jim and I paired up on a Marine who'd been hit by a large shrapnel fragment right above his knee, suffering the now-familiar supracondylar fracture, this time with the added blessing of a severed femoral artery. As we worked to explore his wound, remove shrapnel, and find both ends of the damaged artery, Captain Lea walked into the OR, as he was fond of doing.

"Say, Brief, Lockhart, whatcha guys got here?"

We explained the case, and pointed to the x-rays on the viewbox.

"Nice," continued the Skipper, "no live grenade in there, right?"

"No way, boss," quipped Lockhart. "No live grenades allowed at First Med since Dave Lewis went home!"

We all laughed.

"How do you plan to fix the fracture, Brief?"

"Ninety degree blade plate with eight cortical screws, as soon as my distinguished colleague here clamps off both ends of the artery."

"Kind of similar to your mamasan case at Clinique Phuoc Thieu, no?"

I felt goose bumps. I never spoke to anyone about my work there.

"Whoa, Skipper, how do *you* know about my cases at CPT?"

"Well, you know, I find out a lot about Danang goings-on from my friend Dr. Hoenlein."

Like the rest of Hootch 8, I knew about the Skipper's "friendship" with Dr. Hoenlein, a rather poorly kept secret.

"Who's Dr. Hoenlein?" I lied, as I propped the whole extremity up on bolsters and made a ten-inch lateral incision in the lower half of the thigh to expose the fractured femur.

"Anneliese Hoenlein is chief physician on the German hospital ship, and she knows everybody in town. She told me you work closely with Sister Agatha when you volunteer at CPT."

"Sister Aggie is a great worker," I added cautiously. "She's a major asset in that place."

"She apparently told Anneliese about the two mamasan fractures you treated with the same plate. Cool stuff, Brief."

I hammered the blade part of the device across the femoral condyles about an inch above the knee joint, until the plate part lined up with the shaft of the femur. With Lockhart's help, I then reduced the fracture fragments anatomically, and held the whole thing together with a Lowman clamp.

"Very good, Brief, very fast," joked the Skipper. "Faster than a speeding Dave Lewis!"

"Actually, Skipper, I envy Lewis," I said, driving in my cortical screws. "A mixture of admiration and envy."

"Why envy him? For his Navy Cross?"

I shook my head.

"For his courage. I've been wondering if I would've shown the guts of a Lewis if it'd been me in the OR that day."

"No question in my mind, you would have done the same thing."

"Nice of you to say, Skipper, but I have my doubts."

My ORIF was done. I tested it by raising the leg and flexing the knee a couple of times. It seemed solid. Lockhart took over, and began harvesting his saphenous vein graft in the upper thigh.

"And besides," continued the Skipper, "that stunt you pulled at CPT, whacking the plate out of one femur and sticking it into another, that showed plenty of guts."

"Yeah, well," I said with a sigh, "it didn't turn out so great, did it?"

"Maybe not," the Skipper said as Lockhart measured and prepared his graft, "but seems to me you had little choice. You took a calculated risk and showed plenty of intestinal fortitude. No need to envy Lewis's courage, Brief. You've got plenty of guts yourself."

I was grateful for the Skipper's words. Yet, at the same time, I couldn't help wondering how much he knew about me and Sister Aggie.

Lockhart had reversed his graft and was beginning to suture it in place as I retracted for him.

"Brief," said the Skipper, "how're you getting on with Kaufmann?"

"Fair, Skipper, we don't talk much. When we're in the OR together on a case, it's cordial but cool. As you probably know, after the fragging incident, he apologized, I accepted, and we shook hands, but…I guess the damage was done. He doesn't hang out in Hootch 8 much."

"You know," continued the Skipper as Lockhart kept suturing the graft in place with closely spaced silk stitches, "that whole business about you being Jewish and all, it brought back fond memories."

"Funny, Skipper," quipped Lockhart without missing a beat, "you don't look Jewish!"

"I'm not," laughed the Skipper, "but my roommate in medical school was. Norman Reis, from Chicago. What a fine, great character. Honorable, hardworking, and teller of some of the best jokes I ever heard."

"Where is Dr. Reis now?" I asked.

"Norman Reis is an orthopod like you, a little older, of course. We stayed in touch for a number of years and if memory serves, he is now chief of orthopedics at St. Albans Naval Hospital in Queens, NY."

"Are you kidding me?" I said. "St. Albans is where I am requesting to be assigned when I return from Nam! It's the closest naval hospital to New York City, my hometown."

"Small world, eh?" the Skipper said. "I'll write to him and tell him about you. I'll tell him to kick your ass a little too."

I laughed. By then, Lockhart was nearly finished with his grafting procedure, completing his last row of fine silk sutures in the distal arterial connection.

"Say, Lockhart," said the Skipper, "Do you hear from Rubino at all?"

"Yes, sir," answered Lockhart. "Crumley corresponds with him and it seems he's okay, although his hearing continues to be a problem. He is apparently completing his military obligation at the Naval Station Great Lakes medical facility and he's thrilled to be assigned to the Chicago area, reunited with his wife and family. I'll tell Crumley you asked, Skipper."

"Changing the subject, Captain," I said, "I have a question for you."

"Shoot," he replied.

"Those cool tiger shorts you always wear... are they standard issue?"

"They're not. In fact, a tailor I know in Danang made them for me. Would you like a pair?"

"No thank you, Skipper, I was just curious."

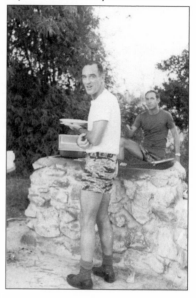

The graft was done. Lockhart released the distal clamp, then the proximal one. Blood began to flow through the restored, grafted artery. What a beautiful sight! The graft bulged a little under the pressure but did not leak, as the sutures held perfectly. Lockhart then checked the dorsalis pedis pulse, which was strong. I raised the leg and flexed the knee again to test my ORIF: it held.

Capt. Lea relaxing in his tiger shorts

We were done, and the Skipper excused himself, complimenting us on our job. We irrigated the wounds, then closed both incisions together, Lockhart closing the medial one and me closing the lateral one, with corpsman Mondello assisting us both.

I thought to myself what a great CO the Skipper was, always fair, always protecting and bolstering his men. It occurred to me that if we were foot soldiers instead of doctors, Captain Lea would be the kind of leader we would blindly follow into battle, no questions asked.

Chapter Twenty-Five

Short-Timer

June rolled by with steady incoming casualties – and frequent nighttime attacks on our compound. The low-crawl into the bunker had practically become a nightly routine. By July 1970, with a little over six weeks left in-country, I was a "short-timer." My short-timer's calendar, a Vargas drawing of an unclad female torso divided into a hundred puzzle pieces with the lowest numbers in strategic places, was beginning to fill up impressively: my daily fill-ins were approaching the pubis, and the breasts were surrounded.

It was time to start thinking about going back to CONUS, back to the world, back to my family. Thoughts ran through my head. What kind of welcome would I be greeted with? Would my homecoming be anti-climactic? Would I be elated or depressed?

In mid-August I received my orders to return home. I was to report to the Danang airport on August 20 at 0930. Imagine that, only 359 days total in Nam! I was getting a six day "huss," a whole six days short of the mandatory year in-country.

On the eve of my departure, Hootch 8 held a party for me, where I had ample chance to say goodbye to everyone: Killjoy, Lockhart, Bardenheier, Gregersen, Alafriz, Mir, and Rashti, as well as corpsmen

Radcliffe and Mondello. Crumley, Widmeyer, and Whitney had already rotated out over the past few weeks. Other pals and colleagues came by to shake hands and share stories, even Kaufmann. Several men gave me their parents' phone numbers to call when I got home. One guy asked me to take money for his girlfriend in Canton, Ohio. I promised him I'd mail her a check.

We laughed, drank, listened to music, and reminisced. We even took turns reading from the "Lens Cleaning Kit" we had originally bought for Rubino's underwater camera. At the back of the box were instructions in two languages: Japanese, and a hilarious broken English which never failed to amuse us. In fact, the lens cleaning kit, together with other stuff like Cuc's notes requesting a day off, and Parker's letter of complaint after we painted his hootch pink, had been compiled into a small dossier jokingly dubbed "The Hootch 8 Scriptures," with which I had been entrusted.

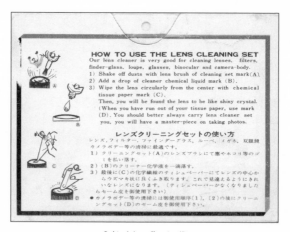

Rubino's Lens Cleaning Kit

The evening of camaraderie passed quickly, and suddenly it was time to go. I was packed and ready, with my big duffle stenciled BRIEF in large white letters, already sitting near the hootch door. At 0730, I stood in the Skipper's office dressed in summer khakis, my service cap perched at a slight angle, my shoes shined.

"Brief," said Captain Lea, leaning forward to shake my hand, "I'm glad to see you go, but I'm not happy to see you go. You did good by First Med. You did your duty, you did not cut corners, you showed up every time and every place we needed you to show up. So for a job well done, you have my gratitude and my admiration."

"Thank you, sir," I replied. "It's been an honor and a privilege to work under your command."

"Although once in a while," he continued, "you got into a bit of a pickle, but you managed to come out alright and handled yourself just fine. Congratulations on being assigned to St. Albans Naval Hospital, where I'm sure you'll get on splendidly with my friend Norman Reis. I've written him about you, and he'll be expecting your arrival there in September as soon as you're done with your three weeks' furlough. So goodbye, Godspeed, and I'll just say this: Brief, you may not be the best orthopedic surgeon I have ever worked with, but you're certainly the funniest."

He stood and shook my hand.

"Captain, knowing how stingy you are with compliments, I much appreciate your words, and I have this to say to you: you may not be the funniest CO I've ever worked with, but you're certainly the fairest."

He laughed, and after a final handshake I turned to leave. As I got to the door, I heard:

"Oh, one more thing Brief, I've got something for you."

I turned around and saw him pull open his top drawer. Then he came around his desk and handed me a small package wrapped in brown paper. It felt soft.

"Just one request, do not open this till you get home."

"Thank you, sir."

I snapped him a salute and walked out.

At 0800, I caught the shuttle vehicle to the airport. I turned around in my seat and watched First Med get smaller and smaller, then disappear around the corner behind a sunlit cloud of dust.

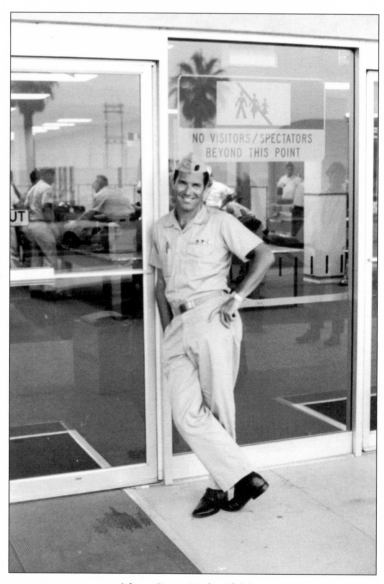

At Danang Airport waiting for my flight home

Chapter Twenty-Six

Flight of Dreams

Wearing jungle fatigues and dark glasses, I sat in a wheelchair pushed by my mother. She wheeled me past large swinging doors into the OR, where my patient was waiting for me, already under anesthesia. Sonny Alafriz stood at the head of the table wearing a sad smile. The patient was a double amputee with smoking stumps bleeding and ragged, reeking of blood. I went to reach for my instruments, then looked down in shock, as both my hands were missing, cut off at the wrists. Suddenly, I realized why the dark glasses: I was also blind.

I woke up with a start, sweating in my airplane seat, having drifted off to sleep after a couple glasses of wine. We were halfway to Hawaii, our stopover. The flight was full of returning GIs who seemed happy and boisterous, but I felt neither. I missed my pals, my patients, and my work. I missed the familiar chaos and frantic pace of First Med, with doctors and corpsmen hustling about every which way. I missed the Clinique Phuoc Thieu, the cadence of the mamasans gliding along the roadsides deftly balancing their heavy shoulder loads, wearing their black silk pants and pointy straw hats, some of them flashing us their black-toothed smiles. I missed the Vietnam lingo like *bookoo, tee tee, di di mau,* in-country, Charlie, even frag, knowing I'd never hear those words again. I missed watching the black GIs exchanging their bumpety-bump handshakes using hands, fists, elbows, shoulders, even hips, handshakes we in Hootch 8 had adopted as our own. I missed the incessant chopper noise, the fuck you lizard, and the entire bittersweet culture of being an American serviceman in Nam.

As I fluctuated in and out of sleep, dozing on and off, thousands of images flashed before me: patients, Crumley's guitar, Tokyo, blood, amputees, OR explosions, ROK Marines, and Hootch 8 laughter.

After a six-hour layover in Honolulu, we continued on to San Francisco. I had more dreams, more flashes of recollection, and sporadic exchanges with other returning servicemen. The flight attendants were solicitous if not overly friendly, an early hint of what awaited us back home.

On the afternoon of August 22, 1970, we touched down in San Francisco. I walked off the plane and set foot on the tarmac. I was home, my year in Vietnam was over.

Chapter Twenty-Seven

Coming Home

Upon arriving back in the US on that August day, I immediately called my parents in New York, both of whom wept with joy, as did my brother Ben and my sister Renee. When they asked when I'd be flying back east, I informed them I needed to be debriefed by the Navy for several days. While this was partially true, the reality was that I intended to spend some time in San Diego with my friend Frieda. I had written to her several weeks before leaving Nam and she had warmly extended an invitation to stop by on my return.

Undeniably, it was a relief to be back on US soil, safe from mosquitoes, malaria, VC rockets, monsoons, mass casualties, choppers, small ants, and the smell of blood. Frieda, my last contact before shipping out in 1969, was mature and calm, open and nurturing, eager to help welcome me back into the world. She'd always been something of a hippie peacenik, but I guess she felt sorry for me. I was not the same man she'd seen one year earlier.

After four wonderful days with her, I flew home to New York. I felt ambivalent, torn between relief at being home in one piece, and missing my life in Hootch 8. Walking the familiar streets of New York, I was easily pegged as a returning veteran because of my short military haircut. There were snide remarks, dirty looks, people spitting on the ground. Not once did I hear "welcome home," or "glad to have you back." Not once did I see a friendly wave or a thumbs up.

Several times a night, I awoke with recurring flashes of amputees, bleeding soldiers, helicopters, and always that smell of blood. On several occasions, I was horrified to recognize my amputee patients as Crumley, Whitney, or Alafriz, causing me to wake up in a sweat. Other nights I was revisited by the nightmare of my mother pushing me in a wheelchair, both my hands cut off at the wrists.

Once, I dreamt Kaufmann and I were fighting in a ring wearing boxing gloves, surrounded by a crowd of laughing and jeering GIs. Kaufmann clearly had the upper hand, sneering at me and wearing a triumphant grin as he pounded my face again and again until I went down in humiliating defeat, blood everywhere. My head slammed down on the canvas with such force that I woke up, out of breath and soaking wet, thinking my perspiration was blood.

A veil of melancholy fell over me. Coupled with the nightmares, the hostility I encountered drove me into a depression. As there existed no organized psychological support for "healthy" returning war veterans in 1970, I had nowhere to turn. While I never expected to be greeted with parades, banner-waving crowds, or welcome home parties, neither did I expect to be made to feel like I was personally responsible for the war. Everywhere I went I was treated with coldness, even contempt.

One Friday evening in synagogue, my parents' rabbi asked me to say a few words about my experiences in Vietnam. I accepted reluctantly and spoke for about ten minutes, after which the congregation stayed around for coffee and cake. A few people came up to thank me, then one man walked over and, in front of my parents, casually announced, "You know, I have long thought that you Vietnam veterans are an affront to the American people."

What could I say? I just walked away.

On my third day back in New York, I called Phil Neufeld, my old friend who had once advised me to run to Canada.

"Paul, nice to have you back! How are you?"

"Tired, a little depressed, but I'm back. Remember you predicted I'd get my ass shot off? Well, glad to report it's intact. My mind … not so great. But how are you, Phil? Haven't heard from you in a while. Everything okay?"

"Yeah, well, a lot's happened here, you know …"

"I understand, life goes on. So let's get together, we'll pop a couple of corks?"

"Well, okay, but …"

Phil seemed hesitant.

"But what Phil? Something wrong?"

"No, nothing's wrong. But I need to tell you something."

"Tell me what, Phil? You're holding back."

"Paul, I'm married."

"Married? Phil, that's great, absolutely wonderful! I'm thrilled for you. So tell me, who's the lucky girl, anyone I know?"

"Yes."

"Really, who? Who is it? Tell me!"

"Marina," he said quietly.

"Marina? My … that Marina?"

"Yes. We were married six months ago. Sorry about the silence, but we both felt bad for you, and a little guilty, what with you being away at war and all …"

I was somewhat shocked by the news, not hurt so much as surprised.

"Congratulations to both of you," I said, "and sincere best wishes."

An awkward silence followed. I now understood why they had both stopped writing sometime last winter. I realized I had no hold on Marina and she owed me nothing, but I wished they had let me know earlier. Our friendship was yet another Vietnam casualty, as I never saw either of them again.

With the passing weeks, my mood began to improve somewhat, and my nightmares became less frequent. My family and a handful of doctor friends – Enrique Ergas, Ben Mizrachy, and Stuart Ring – were supportive and gave generously of their time and attention. I rented a lovely one-bedroom apartment on East 78th Street, furnished it, and began reacquainting myself with civilian clothing and food. My nucleus of good friends rallied around me, inviting me out and helping me regain a sense of normalcy.

I was returned to active military duty that September at St. Albans Naval Hospital in Queens, New York, where I was quickly reminded of the quiet, structured calm of a stateside hospital. There were nurses in starched uniforms, scheduled clinics, elective surgeries, and silent hallways. Not a chopper in sight, no blood spurting from unexpected places, no staff rushing around rolling wounded Marines into surgery with IV bottles held high. It all had the feel of medicine in slow motion.

Just as the Skipper had told me back at First Med, Dr. Norman Reis, the chief of orthopedics, was indeed a gentleman as well as a superbly trained doctor. For a change, he seemed impressed with my service in Vietnam, and we struck up a close friendship.

Meanwhile, it became clear that I had somehow lost my zest for the bachelor life. The partying, the dating, the nonstop frenzied reveling in the sexual revolution – it all seemed childish to me now. I understood that I had come home an older and more introspective man, with a newfound seriousness. Was it the pain and carnage of Vietnam? Had my year at war imparted an understanding of death and an appreciation of life that I had not had before? Whatever the reason, for the first time, I began to entertain the prospect of settling down, much to the delight of my parents, who had long feared I was a confirmed bachelor.

In December 1970 I was notified that the Navy had embarked on a cost-reduction austerity campaign, which included early discharges for personnel returning from combat duty. I was offered the option of an early honorable discharge without delay, along with written confirmation that my military obligation was now fully satisfied. What a huss! Without a moment's hesitation, I signed the necessary papers and found myself released from the Navy, suddenly free as a bird.

The timing was auspicious, as I was planning to take the exam for board certification in orthopedic surgery that spring. Unexpectedly, I found myself with a full three months to devote to catching up on orthopedic literature, which was a huge relief. Vietnam hadn't exactly been conducive to study, and I'd fallen behind in my reading.

I began by mapping out a detailed study plan, then went straight to work. Waking at seven in the morning, I would read, study, review, and memorize until eight at night. Knowing I had some eighty-five days of study before me, I carefully divided my time to cover the various orthopedic disciplines, such as fractures and trauma, pediatric orthopedics, adult orthopedics, hand surgery, foot and ankle, sports medicine, bone pathology, metabolic diseases, infectious diseases, and arthritis. I reserved daily time for review of orthopedic journals and old board examinations. Once a week, I went food shopping and typically ate at home alone, cooking simple stuff myself. I kept in touch with family and friends during the evenings, though I rarely went out.

I took the board exam in Chicago in March 1971 and was fortunate enough to pass. Now a board certified orthopedic surgeon, I began to look for work, still nursing a lingering depression, which resurfaced after the focused distraction of three months of solid study.

One evening in April, my good friend Ben Mizrachy knocked on my door and told me I needed a break.

"Why don't we take a week at Club Med in Martinique?"

"No thank you, Ben," I replied. "I prefer to sit here and mope. I'm in no mood to socialize much."

Ben then produced two tickets to Martinique and said in his singsong South African accent, "As you wish, Paul. I'll just have to chalk up your ticket as a loss, won't I?"

How could I disappoint my friend? We left the following week and arrived in sunny Club Med, where I promptly fell ill with a nasty case of the flu. Lying on the beach the following day wrapped in a blanket and shivering with fever, I was surprised to see an attractive, older woman walk over and sit next to me.

"What's wrong?" she said in a soft European accent.

"I'm sick and I feel awful, please don't come too close."

"Oh, not to worry. I'm here with my doctor husband and we always travel with lots of medicine. I'll get you well in no time."

Ellie and Ed Kahan doctored me with antibiotics, decongestants, and aspirin, and within forty-eight hours, I was nearly recovered. Ben and I hung out with them for the rest of our vacation and we became friends. Ellie took a particular liking to me.

"You seem to be a nice young man," she told me one day, "so I'm going to get you married. We have lots of friends back in Mamaroneck with adorable daughters."

And so it began. Upon my return to New York, I was fixed up with a string of young women, each one pretty, smart, and educated. But there was no chemistry, no spark, nothing. After several of these blind dates, Ellie called me up.

"You know, Paul, you seem to be a difficult case, too much for me to handle. But I still have hope for you, so I'm going to hand you over to the care of my daughter-in-law."

Now Betsy Kahan, who was a graduate student in psychology at Columbia University, took her turn at me. I treated each date nicely, politely, trying to be a perfect gentleman, but I had no interest. Betsy called me in desperation.

"Look, Paul, I don't know what to do, my bag of tricks is empty. I do have one last suggestion for you. She's a Ph.D. student at Columbia with me and she seems nice, although I don't know her well. And that's about it, my friend. Her name is Rochelle Frankel."

I called Rochelle the following day, a Monday. Her response was cool, as Betsy had probably told her I was difficult, but she agreed to a date later that week. Due to my recent run of failed blind dates, and given Betsy's less-than-enthusiastic description of Rochelle Frankel, I was prepared for another disappointment when I rang her doorbell on Thursday, January 6, 1972.

The door opened and there she stood, wearing a faint smile, a brown beret, brown corduroy slacks, and a thick-knit orange sweater. She was slender yet well proportioned, and very pretty. Actually, she was beautiful. I started going down my bachelor's mental checklist... *nothing wrong... how can there be nothing wrong?... alert... alert...*

I couldn't take my eyes off her. I helped her on with her coat, and we began walking the Columbia neighborhood as we talked. We dropped into the West End Bar on Broadway, where we sat at a quiet corner table facing each other. She ordered a Bloody Mary and I, a Brandy Alexander. We talked and talked. I believe it was love at first sight for both of us, that rarest of thunderbolts supposedly only found in romance novels.

I asked her out the following evening. She said yes and we were together every evening thereafter except for the following Monday, when we both had previously arranged dates, which, for whatever reason, we felt obligated to keep.

Our romance progressed at a dizzying pace, and we announced our engagement in April to the shock and consternation of my friends, who were convinced I'd never marry, especially since I had returned from Vietnam with a bruised psyche. But Betsy Kahan, our *shadchan*, her mother Ellie Kahan, and our respective parents, were spinning with delight.

I never formally proposed, which hardly seemed necessary. We had already committed to each other on that fateful evening of January 6, 1972. Or perhaps it was the next evening. To this day, we still celebrate two anniversaries: January 6 and September 3, 1972, our wedding day. Forty years, four children, and two grandchildren later, it is still love at first sight every time I see her.

On October 6, 1973, barely one year after our wedding, Rochelle and I were sitting in synagogue during Yom Kippur services when we saw someone walk up to the rabbi and whisper in his ear. Visibly taken aback, the rabbi interrupted his sermon and announced that war had broken out in the Middle East. Israel was under attack on multiple fronts; the Yom Kippur War had begun.

As a murmur of alarm rumbled through the congregation, I whispered to Rochelle that I'd like to go to Israel to help, and would she come with me. Without a moment's hesitation, she said yes and we ran home. I put in an emergency call to Dr. Meyer Makin, chief of orthopedics at Hadassah Hospital in Jerusalem. In 1969, several months before leaving for Vietnam, I had done a three-month rotation at Hadassah as part of my residency training. There, I had befriended a number of Israeli orthopods, including the influential and highly respected Dr. Makin.

"Yes," he said when I finally reached him in the middle of the night, "we need you. Your experience in combat orthopedics is recent, while ours goes back to the Six Day War in 1967. Come right over."

"But Dr. Makin," I replied, "how can we get there? El Al Israel Airlines is only accepting returning Israeli citizens, soldiers, and diplomats. I am none of the above."

"Not to worry, I'll arrange for tickets via diplomatic pouch."

The next day, a courier delivered an envelope containing three airline tickets to Israel. Why three? I'll never know. I immediately called my best friend, Chilean orthopedist Enrique Ergas. I informed Enrique that he was coming to Israel with us at Dr. Makin's invitation. We would be serving as surgical volunteers at Hadassah, most likely for the duration of the war.

"What?" came his bewildered reply. "You must be crazy! You just came back from a war, and now you're running to another one, and you want me to go with you? No way!"

"Enrique, I'm going, Rochelle is going, and we need your skills, so you're going too. Pack your bag, we're picking you up at 6 A.M. on the way to the airport. See you in the morning."

He came with us. The El Al Boeing 747 was packed with homebound Israelis as well as a good number of American medical volunteers like us, all rushing off to do their part in the Yom Kippur War.

But that's a whole other story.

Chapter Twenty-Eight

An Argument You Cannot Win

While most nightmares are dreams, some happen in real life and can haunt a person forever. One such nightmare occurred in 1973 and torments me to this day.

One of the principal medical lessons I learned in Vietnam was the proper handling of limb injuries in which there was both a major fracture and a damaged artery. Coordinated teamwork between the orthopedic and vascular specialists is vital. As we'd been taught back in FSMS at Pendleton, such cases require that the fracture be fixed first, before the vascular repair graft. Reversing that sequence is considered a grave error; motion between the sharp bony fragments may stretch, tear, or obstruct the arterial repair, leading to loss of circulation, gangrene, and eventual amputation.

In the summer of 1973, only a few weeks after starting my orthopedic practice in Rockland County, New York, and joining the staff of the local hospital, I answered a duty call to the ER for a patient with a supracondylar fracture of the femur. The injury, caused by a truck tire blowout, was open, and the patient had no pedal pulse, having apparently suffered a damaged femoral artery.

As I drove to the hospital, I found myself wishing that Jim Lockhart, my old pal and a great vascular surgeon, would be there. When I got to the ER, a mere fifteen minutes after being called, the x-rays showed a typical transverse supracondylar fracture with slight displacement. Easy, I thought, quickly assessing the films and envisioning ORIF with a ninety-degree blade-plate and eight or ten screws. Familiar stuff.

But when I asked the nurse where the patient was, she informed me he was already in the OR.

"Why?" I inquired. "I'm on first ortho call, I came as soon as I was called, so what's he doing in the OR?"

"Oh," she replied casually, "Dr. Stoltz was on first trauma call and took him to the OR a while ago."

A feeling of dread mixed with resentment came over me. Stoltz, chief of surgery, had been called first and took the patient right up to work on his open wound and address his arterial injury. I rushed right upstairs, put on scrubs, and walked into the OR, where Stoltz was working away, assisted by his new junior partner, a man about my age.

"Brief, you're the new orthopedist, right?"

"Yes, sir, I am," I replied.

"What do you think of the x-rays?" asked Dr. Stoltz.

"Displaced supracondylar femur, sir, needs fixation with a compression blade-plate."

"Yeah, well, not now it doesn't. I'm doing an arterial graft first, so when I'm done, you can put his leg in pin traction. It's too late now to think of a plate, or whatever you call it. If you do that now, you'll damage my graft with all the pulling and banging around you orthopods are known for."

"Sir, with all due respect," I replied, "I believe the ORIF should be done first, before the vascular work. Leaving this man in traction without solid fracture fixation will allow the bone fragments to move around each time he turns in bed or contracts his muscles. And this will damage your vascular repair."

Stoltz stopped working and turned to me, angry and red-faced.

"Now look here, young man. I was called first, this is my case, and I believe I'm doing the right thing here. How dare you question my judgment! Do you know how many years I've been doing this? And where were you this morning, anyway?"

"Sir, I came as soon as I was called, only to find the patient already in the OR. I can tell you that in the military, where we treated a large number of these cases, we were strongly indoctrinated in the proper surgical staging for the patient's best interests, and…"

"Stop right there!" yelled Stoltz. "This is the United States, not Vietnam or wherever the hell you were. I'll have no more of this and if you don't mind, I'd like to finish my operation. In recovery you can put his leg in traction. Now please go."

I left the room furious and promptly called the chief of orthopedics, and explained the entire situation to him. Dr. Edward Leahey was an older man who was smart and authoritative but also diplomatic.

"Look, Paul," he advised, "you are in a no-win situation here. This Stoltz is a tyrant and a megalomaniac, and he'd rather die than take a suggestion from a young attending like you, right or wrong. I've had my own run-ins with him and he's never wrong, even when he's wrong."

"So what should I do here, Dr. Leahey? This bothers the hell out of me, and I've got a sickening feeling this poor patient is going to lose his leg."

"I agree with you," he replied. "But now that Stoltz is in the middle of doing his graft, what do you expect him to do? Take it down and let you take over? And worst of all, even if he yielded and let you take over to fix the fracture now, there's no guarantee the poor devil won't lose his leg anyway. Then you'll really be up the creek, because Stoltz will not hesitate to put the blame on you. You've been here all of a month and that could ruin you."

"So what do I do?"

"Let it go," he said. "Do as he says, drive a pin in his upper tibia, and put the leg in Russell traction. If the leg is lost, at least Stoltz can't blame *you* for it. Believe me, I've dealt with this guy before and this is an argument you cannot win."

I felt crushed. But I realized that Dr. Leahey was probably right. I was caught in a no-win situation and so was the patient.

For the next three weeks, I struggled daily, adjusting the traction, taking multiple x-rays, and watching in desperation as the pedal pulses grew faint, then disappeared. The leg began to turn colors: first white, then red, then purplish. During the third week, two toes turned black, signaling the arrival of gangrene. The leg was dead. We amputated above the knee twenty-two days after the injury.

I was devastated and lost many nights of sleep. Although Dr. Stoltz was clearly to blame, I blamed myself too. Why had I not stood up to him more forcefully? Why had I not made a scene, jumping up and down, yelling and screaming until I got my way? How would Dave Lewis have handled this? In Vietnam, he had stood up to the Skipper and prevailed. Why couldn't I? Was this simply another sign that I lacked courage? I couldn't shake the thought that I had failed to heed the most important lesson I'd learned in Vietnam.

Chapter Twenty-Nine

Memorial

After the Washington D.C. Vietnam Memorial was unveiled in 1983, I made a concerted effort to visit often. I missed a number of years, but I've been there over a dozen times. Each time, I feel inspired by the elegant simplicity and somber melancholy of the long, black granite structure which bears the names of the 58,267 men and women who fell in Vietnam.

Actually, the wall always looks green to me, as the grass surrounding it on all sides is reflected in its shiny surface. I bring flowers and lay them down somewhere along the wall, choosing a spot at random which looks empty. I walk from the thin angled point only a few inches high on one end, past the middle where the wall stands ten feet tall, to the other end, where it tapers off again. The wall starts out thin, then gets larger and larger, a bit like the war itself.

I look at individual names but do not recognize them because, as I mentioned before, I did not record the names of my patients (except for one) and anyway, the KIAs did not come through our hospital, but went directly to the Graves Unit for identification, family notification, and transfer home.

When I visited on the morning of May 15, 2001, accompanied by my daughter Amanda who was then fourteen, I had no reason to think this visit would be different from any other. We walked the length of the wall, back and forth, and Amanda put down the flowers. We admired the memorial statues of the Three Infantrymen and the Women's Memorial, all beautiful, all sad. Then, as we began to walk away, I noticed for the first time the directory volume at the western end of the wall. I had a thought: Should I look him up? Is he dead or alive? Since my return in 1970, I had written Donald Duffy on three occasions, never receiving a reply. I thought for a moment and said to Amanda, "Just a minute, sweetheart. I need to look up something."

I walked to the directory, my heart beating hard. Duc...Dud... Duf...there he was: "Duffy, Donald b.1950 d.1971. Lance Corporal, USMC, First Marine Division, Kimberly, Idaho." My heart sank, my vision blurred. I felt shivers. Holding my daughter's hand, I began to walk away, then sank to a sitting position on the grass. A second later, my head fell into my hands and I began to sob uncontrollably. My patient was dead, my mind was spinning, and my heart was broken. How many times could my heart break? I felt as if I had lost a brother or worse, a son. Pictures of Donald flashed in my head: the surgery, the bandages, the weeks spent caring for him and conversing with him.

How had he died? Had he succumbed to some late infection? Had his kidneys failed as a late result of the dozens of transfusions, or had he simply taken his own life? These questions raced through my mind as I continued to sob, overcome with a sadness and grief I had not felt since my father's death in 1980. Amanda, not knowing what to make of this, simply sat there with her arm around me, her head on my shoulder, and began crying too. A few people surrounded us and one woman handed me tissues, while a longhaired veteran wearing a faded jungle fatigue jacket sat down quietly beside me.

I don't remember how long we sat there. When my crying finally stopped, I told Amanda the story of Donald Duffy, a story I had not told anyone before. Tears rolled down her cheeks and I wiped them. Eventually, we stood up in the morning sun and hand in hand, walked to join my wife Rochelle, who awaited us at the Smithsonian with our other children: Andy, Joanna, and James. As Amanda and I traversed the Washington Mall, cherry blossoms all around us, I remembered sitting at Donald's bedside, talking to him as he scribbled answers on his notepad. For me, the misery of the war knew no end.

Chapter Thirty

Reunion

I kept loosely in touch with several pals from Hootch 8, but never actually got together with any of them until years later, upon receiving the following letter from Crumley, dated San Francisco, October 2, 1984.

"Here's the scoop:

The First Medical Battalion Reunion/Bash is scheduled for Monday night, October 22, at 7:00 P.M. The location is the Board Room at the Bohemian Club, 624 Taylor Street. It is about two blocks from Union Square, and the entrance is between Post and Sutter Streets. We'll have a nice private room where the gooks' rockets won't fall.

I'll have a Super 8 movie projector, and Kodak Carousel projector, so bring your flicks of whatever kind. I figure that at least one hour of cocktails will be necessary, then a good can of C-rats, then we can pretend we're at the O-Club watching round-eyes, or go to the vil.

I'm still waiting to hear back from Jim Lea, and haven't located Whitney yet, maybe they went to Australia together on R & R, to retrieve Parker's dildo. Would appreciate you calling Widmeyer in Roanoke VA and demanding that he be here. Anyone else you can

think of, give them a call... and be sure that they let me know. See
you then... for mid-rats.
> *Signed: Lifer Rog."*

And so, a couple weeks later, at seven o'clock, I walked into San Francisco's Bohemian Club, a sumptuous turn-of-the-century institution boasting the likes of Ronald Reagan and Gerald Ford as members. When I entered the private hall, decorated with chandeliers, brocade cloth walls, classic paintings, and lush Persian rugs, I was thrilled to see a number of "Hootcheighters" already in attendance. Within fifteen minutes, everyone had arrived: Crumley, Widmeyer, Whitney, Alafriz, Captain Lea, Rubino, Blumberg, Kilroy, Cave, Bardenheier, and other First Med dignitaries.

It was wonderful, with about twenty five men talking, laughing, hugging, back slapping, and wiping an occasional tear. Roger Crumley had arranged everything, from the luxurious hall (he was a member and had met President Reagan), to the audio-visuals, the food, the drink, and the program. Everything was perfect, down to the music. Roger had made a tape which played on a huge boom box, pumping out our favorite tunes from Nam – The Beatles' "Let It Be," "Hey Jude," and "Eleanor Rigby," as well as Hootch 8 classics like "People Are Strange" by The Doors, Steppenwolf's "Born to be Wild," and Procol Harum's "Whiter Shade of Pale."

After two hours of cocktailing, reminiscing, and comparing notes, we all sat down at a long table with a floor-length white tablecloth, Crumley and the Skipper at either end. I sat somewhere near the middle with a good view of everybody. The dinner was strictly gourmet, with two marvelous wines poured liberally by white-gloved servers: a smooth, silky 1981 Louis Martini Cabernet Sauvignon, and a delectable 1982 Château Montelena Chardonnay (a later vintage of the famed California white wine which had won the historic 1976 blind tasting in Paris, putting to shame all the great French white burgundies such as Montrachet and Corton-Charlemagne). I had no idea Crumley was such a connoisseur, and complimented him on his selections.

As dinner progressed, Crumley stood up, tapped his glass, and announced:

"Gentlemen, thank you all for joining us to share in some decent

C-rations as well as acceptable grape juice" (laughter). "I certainly appreciate so many of you having gone to great lengths to join us, and I hope a good time is being had by all. I want you to know that behind this door on my right, we have three mamasans who will come out later and do your laundry" (table-banging, hoots, whistles, and laughter). "After dessert, the Sergeant Major will come in and force every one of you to take a CP malaria pill, so prepare to be good and sick with the runs for the next three days" (more laughter). "Paul Brief will then give a slide show on small ants, Widmeyer will show us his muscles, and Killjoy will lead us in a chorus of 'When the Saints Come Marching In.'

"Then, for mid-rats, we will all take a walk to Union Square Park and listen to the fuck you lizard work out" (the laughing, jeering, and cat-whistling reached a crescendo).

"And now, I give you the one, the only, the Skipper: Captain Jim Lea."

He extended his arm to Captain Lea, who stood as we all rose to our feet, clapping, whistling, and cheering. The Skipper gave a cordial thank-you to Crumley for arranging and laboring over the reunion. He also thanked the entire group for attending, telling us with some emotion how honored and privileged he felt for having worked with all of us at First Med.

After another long round of applause and a standing ovation, Crumley stood again and asked each one of us to say something. And so we each took our turns regaling a receptive, wine-soaked crowd about our lives and our work, showing slides of families with smiling children and lovely wives. Some of the speeches and presentations were memorable enough to mention here.

Bob Cave, our general surgeon/chef was practicing in Charleston, South Carolina, and showed us slides of his beautiful home and sizeable boat. Then he pulled out a copy of his recently published cookbook *Caveman Cuisine*, which he proudly passed around. An impressive tome of some 275 pages, complete with mouth-watering photos and countless recipes, he also passed around a sheet of paper for all our addresses, promising to send copies to each and every one of us.

Sonny Alafriz told us how he'd settled in Phoenix and started a large anesthesia group practice, servicing a number of hospitals.

"I'd like to show you some pictures of my babies," he said and proceeded to flash slide after slide of magnificent homes, commercial buildings, apartment complexes, and shopping malls. It seemed Sonny had invested heavily in real estate, and as I found out later in a private chat, had become enormously wealthy. It couldn't have happened to a nicer guy.

Every presentation was laced with self-deprecatory remarks, and greeted with rowdy comments from the bleachers.

Dave Whitney was practicing orthopedics in Washington state and frequently volunteered his skills for multiple charitable medical missions to Kenya, Ghana, Zaire, and other African countries.

Crumley combined a private ENT practice with academic medicine in San Francisco, and was apparently on track to becoming department chairman at UCSF Medical Center, if only he could manage to conceal his rowdy past from the academic Brahmins. Then he turned somewhat serious, pulled out a newspaper clipping, and began reading: "*San Francisco Chronicle*, May 18, 1982..."

Apparently, the local police had received multiple complaints about one Robert Kaufmann from his neighbors, as he had repeatedly been blaring Nazi martial music from large speakers installed in his backyard. The police arrived to find him drunk, disorderly, and combative. Eventually convicted of resisting arrest and assaulting a police officer, Kaufmann received a prison sentence and had his medical license revoked.

A murmur of surprise buzzed through the room, with some heads turning to look at me. Sensing this as a perfect opportunity to keep my mouth shut, I said nothing.

Then Roger deftly restored the mood by announcing, "Now I would like to hear from our very own Leatherman, Bob Widmeyer!"

Widmeyer stood to a round of applause, taking a mock bow as he told us about his sports medicine practice and his beautiful family in Roanoke, his short-sleeved shirt betraying a Schwarzenegger-like musculature. He was greeted with whistles and comments like "Show us your pecs!" and "How about some arm wrestling?" amid raucous laughter.

As the time kept passing and the wine kept flowing, the mood only escalated, so when Blumberg the warrior-dentist stood to speak, he was greeted with shouts of "Open wide!" "Show us your tongue!" and "Hey doc, where's your guns?"

In response, he said: "As you can all note, I can speak again and no, there are no guns tonight. But I did bring this."

He reached into his shirt pocket and produced the A K 47 round Crumley had so expertly removed from his tongue, to wild applause. That thing was huge, like some gigantic suppository, and I had a flash recollection of that unforgettable skull x-ray with the bullet sitting upright in his mouth, clenched between his teeth.

When my turn came, I read from The Hootch 8 Scriptures, including the "Lens Cleaning Kit" instructions and a letter from our old housekeeper Cuc, both of which were greeted with much laughter. Then I put on a semi-serious air, briefly discussing my family, before saying, "Gentlemen, like my good friend Dr. Blumberg, I too brought a Vietnam trophy to show you."

With that, I stood on my chair, stepped onto the table, loosened my belt, and pulled down my zipper. My pants fell around my ankles to wild laughter, and there they were: Captain Lea's tiger shorts. As the applause, catcalls, and whistling grew frantic, the Skipper, himself laughing hard, stood and held his hands out to calm the crowd.

"Gentlemen, let me explain. Late in his tour in Nam, Brief here expressed admiration for my tiger shorts, so on the day he left, I gave them to him in appreciation for his good work."

More laughter and whistling.

"And I must say," he continued, "that I'm impressed they still fit after all these years!"

I pulled up my pants, waited for the laughter to die down, and said: "Not really, Skipper, my tailor had to let them out."

There was more cheering as I walked over and gave him a hug as a belated thank-you for his gift.

But the evening was unquestionably stolen by Paul Rubino. He stood up, and with some emotion, thanked us all for inviting him, for having supported him during his stay at First Med, for being such good friends, and for thinking about him after all these years.

"And now, with your permission, I'd like to take pictures of all of you," he said, snapping pictures all around with the camera that was hanging from his neck as we all applauded. We thought nothing of it, as most of us had brought cameras, when suddenly Paul bent down, lifted up the floor-length tablecloth, and pulled out a plastic bucket filled with water, placing it smack in the middle of the table. Then, before any of us realized what was happening, he pulled the camera from around his neck, and with a deft basketball move, dunked it into the water with a gigantic splash, dousing a number of us sitting in close proximity. It was his Nikonos underwater camera! The place went wild, with guys cheering and laughing so hard I saw a couple of them fall off their chairs. It was complete pandemonium, with half of us wet, and deservedly so.

If ever there were such a thing as comedic retribution, this was it. The man had taken our practical joke and turned it on us in one brilliant move. All the guys came around, laughing, shaking Paul's hand, and patting his back, congratulating him on his good sportsmanship.

I looked at my watch. It was 1:45 A.M. Where had the evening gone? After we all said our goodbyes, with promises to keep in touch, I walked downstairs to find my wife, waiting patiently to walk me the few blocks back to the St. Francis Hotel. She was wise indeed to have come for me, as I could not have managed that walk on my own.

One final, sad footnote about the reunion. The reader will remember my old fried Dick Nottingham, "the Sheriff," whom I mentioned early in the story as someone who had been with me through all of my college, medical, and post-graduate education, ending up with me in Hootch 8. Then I made no further mention of him. It turns out Dick developed a knee problem shortly after we got to Vietnam and was sent home only six weeks after our arrival there. After that, we more or less lost touch, until I sadly learned in 2002 that he had developed a brain tumor and was very ill. Dick Nottingham died in 2004 at the age of sixty-four, leaving behind his wife, three children, and a thriving orthopedic practice.

Epilogue

I t was never my intention to delve into the politics of the Vietnam War, as I wrote this book strictly from the viewpoint of a doctor and half-baked humorist. I realized decades ago that the terrible things I saw in Vietnam, combined with the mind-bending effort demanded of me, could have caused me to tumble off the edge of sanity into a psychotic abyss. What saved me from such a fate was the constant support, comradeship and comic relief generously provided by my First Med friends. It is this paradox, this "tragicomedy" of war, which I wanted to portray.

But as a Vietnam veteran, notwithstanding my reluctance to make political statements, I am pained each time I hear casual remarks like, "We should have never been in Vietnam," or "Vietnam was a pointless war," or worst of all, "Fifty-eight thousand Americans died in Vietnam for nothing."

If one substitutes "Korea" in the above remarks, they end up sounding bizarre, because nobody ever complains that Korea was a pointless war, or that 44,692 American troops died in vain. Why the difference? As I pointed out in these pages, the 58,267 men and women who gave their lives in Vietnam died for essentially the same reason the

44,692 fallen in Korea did, which was an effort, fueled by the Cold War, to stem the tide of communism.

The principal difference between these two wars is that in Korea we won, whereas in Vietnam we lost. After three years of bitter fighting in Korea, the US prevailed, and to this day we maintain a military presence in South Korea, a democratic and prosperous ally, while North Korea remains an impoverished, totalitarian regime. Conversely, in Vietnam, after ten years of a halfheartedly fought conflict, the US withdrew its forces in 1973, leaving the country in the care of the ARVN.

No match for the vastly superior communist NVA forces led by the brilliant General Giap, the feeble ARVN was quickly overrun, leading to the unification of the country under the communist banner in 1975. Yet the loss of the war in Vietnam does not change the fact that it was fought for the same reason as Korea.

In 1989, a mere fourteen years after the fall of Vietnam, the entire Soviet Empire collapsed, the Berlin Wall came down, and the face of communism was changed forever.

My friend Paul Adler, a former Democratic Party County Chairman and an astute political analyst, believes that the collapse of the Soviet Union was not so much a political phenomenon as an economic one. The Soviet economy simply went bankrupt as a result of its overextended reach.

Adler maintains that this economic downfall was the culmination of a process that began with Vietnam. It is no secret that throughout the conflict, which began with French involvement in 1946 and ended with the communist takeover in 1975, North Vietnam was armed, supplied, and financed by the Soviet regime. This enormous financial burden continued into the 1980s as a newly unified and financially strapped communist Vietnam required heavy loans and infrastructural financing. Coupled with other involvements in places like Cuba, Angola, and Afghanistan, this proved to be an unbearable financial burden which hobbled the Soviet economy, culminating in its full financial breakdown.

But if the US became involved in Vietnam as a stand against communism, and if that war eventually brought down the Soviet Empire, did we not, in fact, achieve our goal? And if we achieved our goal, albeit with the appearance of military defeat, did we not ultimately come out victorious?

I realize perhaps better than most how difficult it is to get over the loss of the 58,000, a wound that remains open, as millions of American parents, spouses, children, siblings, relatives, and friends continue to grieve. And that's without counting the hundreds of thousands of physically and mentally injured Vietnam veterans who still live in our midst.

During the 1960s, '70s, and '80s, the media did such a job of demonizing the war and brainwashing the public, that the American psyche suffered a crippling blow from which we have yet to fully recover. Who can forget the footage of frantic Vietnamese storming the US Embassy compound in Saigon on our last day there, desperately trying to board that helicopter as it lifted off? Or the chopper that tumbled off the edge of the aircraft carrier into the ocean? These images of panic and chaos still haunt us.

Vietnam was, and still is, dubbed "a bad war." It was the first war America ever "lost" in its 240-year history. There seems to be a national consensus that no good whatsoever came out of that war, that it had no redeeming value. I beg to differ with most of these statements, believing not only in the justness of the war, but in its ultimate effectiveness in achieving our goal of weakening the Soviet Union. As Adler and some historians have argued, the war was a significant factor in the economic burdens that eventually crippled communism.

It also cannot be ignored that great advances emerged from Vietnam in areas such as medicine and military science. In the medical field, great progress was made on multiple levels. Helicopter medevacs, which had their humble beginnings in Korea, became a precise science in Vietnam and saved countless lives. Wound care made great strides. The use of antibiotics in open, contaminated wounds became highly sophisticated. But perhaps most importantly, the fields of rehabilitation medicine and limb prosthetics saw enormous advances in Vietnam's aftermath, as amputees were enabled to regain a degree of functionality once thought unattainable.

Our understanding of tropical diseases such as malaria, typhoid, and other fevers increased, as did our understanding of parasitic infestations, facilitating treatment and recovery. Rapid deployment and installation of mobile field hospitals reached levels of efficiency previously unheard of. When the medical lessons learned in Vietnam were applied to subsequent conflicts such as Iraq and Afghanistan, the result was improved survival rates for our casualties.

From a military viewpoint, advances in troop mobility, weapon modernization, and equipment computerization emerged in Vietnam. Troop mobility was forever changed by the helicopter, a form of transport which will forever symbolize Vietnam in our collective memory. For the first time in US military history, helicopters were utilized for the quadruple purpose of troop deployment, assault tactics, airlifting of casualties, and heavy equipment transport.

There were numerous occasions when four helicopters would swoop down on a combat area. The larger Chinook would drop off troop reinforcements while the medium-sized Cheyenne, equipped as a flying ambulance, picked up the wounded. Meanwhile, two Huey helicopter gunships circled the area like birds of prey, laying down heavy machine gun and rocket fire on the enemy. From the vantage point of the First Med perimeter, it all resembled an aerial ballet. At night, with tracer bullets streaming red from the helicopter guns, and multi-colored flares lighting up the skies, the scene had the feel of operatic fireworks, complete with the smell of gunpowder and the ear-splitting din. For heavy transport, the huge Sikorskys could lift and relocate trucks, armored personnel carriers (APC), and other equipment previously considered untransportable in a jungle environment.

As for weapon modernization, this was highlighted by the introduction of the M16 as the weapon of choice for US infantry in Vietnam. Highly accurate, light, and reliable, the M16 facilitated troop mobility in a jungle setting. The M60 machine gun, also introduced in Vietnam, was a dramatic improvement over the heavier and slower BAR used in WWII and Korea.

Grenades, thrown by hand during most of WWII and Korea, saw the introduction of the RPG in Vietnam, a major advance in hand-to-hand combat. The M79 was lighter, more accurate, and more effective than earlier grenades, and could be launched from a specialized rifle.

American domination of the Vietnam skies was honed to a supersonic level of sophistication, facilitated by computer advances. The F4 Phantom jet had virtually no opposition in the skies; no Russian aircraft could compete with it. While in WWII a majority of Army Air Force (AAF) casualties were caused by technical malfunction rather than by enemy fire, in Vietnam that ratio was reversed, with almost no losses due to accidental crashes.

Beyond the medical and military advances, I believe we learned an important national lesson in the aftermath of Vietnam. Over the past two decades, it has become clear to most Americans that soldiers returning from a combat zone, regardless of where it is, cannot and must not be mistreated by their fellow citizens. By the early 1990s the mistreatment my Nam buddies and I experienced upon our return had become a source of national shame and embarrassment.

Today, Americans go out of their way to welcome and show respect for Iraq and Afghanistan returnees, a shift we owe to Vietnam. There has also been a growing emphasis on facilitating treatment of PTSD (post traumatic stress disorder) for men and women returning from war zones today, also perhaps a direct effect of the post-Vietnam neglect.

The Vietnam War is still too close historically to draw conclusions about all of its long-term effects. We do not have a bird's eye view of history that allows for full judgment. A good example of that phenomenon is Harry Truman. For over thirty years after his term of office, he was considered a mediocre president, only to enjoy an astonishing turnaround in the mid-1980s, and he is now considered one of the greatest leaders of the twentieth century.

Could our opinion of the Vietnam War eventually undergo such a turnaround? Could the bird's eye view of history, combined with an understanding of the war's positive effects, eventually lead to a newfound appreciation of the American involvement in Vietnam? Adler believes, and I agree, that the contrast between the old demonizing of the war and its potential reversal, constitutes the true paradox of Vietnam.

As a Nam vet with undying empathy and affection for my fellow veterans, I do not believe that the 58,267 died in vain. With time, I trust that they will be seen as the heroes they truly were. It is my sincere hope that all Vietnam vets, living or not, will someday receive the national welcome and appreciation they still await.

Glossary

Adductor magnus: Large muscle located on the inner or medial aspect of the thigh, coursing from the hip to just above the knee.

AKA: Above knee amputation, or above knee amputee.

AK47: Automatic assault weapon favored by Russia and China, supplied to the North Vietnamese army and Vietcong guerillas during the Vietnam War. Also named Kalashnikov, the AK47 became the standard communist weapon in the Vietnam War, just as the M16 was the standard weapon for American forces.

Anatomical reduction: Setting or reducing a fracture so that the fracture fragments fit perfectly or "anatomically."

Anterior: Front of the body or a body part, as opposed to posterior, which is the back of the body or a body part.

ARVN: Army of the Republic of Vietnam, the South Vietnamese armed forces who fought alongside the US against communist North Vietnam. When the US withdrew from Vietnam in 1973, they handed over control of the country to the ARVN forces.

Attending: Attending physician, a doctor who is a legitimate member of a hospital medical staff. Prior to acceptance as an attending physician, the doctor is subject to a thorough review of his/her past record, including education, residency training, Board certification, previous hospital affiliations, and past criminal record, if any.

BAR: Browning automatic rifle, a heavy machine gun in use during WWII and Korea. The BAR was replaced by the M60 machine gun in Vietnam.

Bennett retractor: A cobra-shaped retractor used in pairs, for holding soft tissue away from a bone to facilitate visualization of that bone.

Bentsch gomel: From the Yiddish meaning "Bless Gomel" or recite the Gomel prayer. This prayer of gratitude is recited before the Torah, usually in the presence of a rabbi, by a person who has had a recent brush with death, escaped injury, undergone surgery, or recovered from serious illness.

Betel nut: A grain or seed chewed as a mild stimulant in Asia and the South Pacific, the Betel Nut can cause permanent black discoloration of the teeth. In Vietnam, many older women sported a black-toothed smile.

BKA: Below knee amputation, or below knee amputee.

Black teeth: See Betel Nut

Bookoo: From the French "beaucoup," meaning many, much, very, or a lot. Bookoo was one of many such words incorporated into Vietnamese colloquialism during the French occupation of Vietnam. It was also adopted by American troops.

Brig: Navy term for prison, equivalent to Army stockade. The brig was reserved for Navy or Marine Corps prisoners, not members of the other armed services.

Butterfly fragment: In a long bone fracture such as a femur, the fracture usually consists of two main fragments. However, there is often a third, relatively smaller piece of bone lying adjacent to the major fragments, called a "butterfly fragment."

Bypass graft: A vascular graft usually made up of a length of vein from a patient's lower limb, used to bridge the gap in a damaged or severed artery where there is a length of artery missing. Can also be called "interposition graft."

Charlie: Slang name given to the enemy, usually Vietcong or NVA.

Charoset: A concoction served at the Passover Seder, made of a mixture of apples, nuts, and wine, symbolizing the mortar used by Jews during their enslavement in Egypt.

Clinique Phuoc Thieu: A civilian hospital in Danang where I did weekly volunteer work on Vietnamese civilians, alongside other doctor and nurse volunteers. As most Vietnamese medical personnel had been conscripted into the military, the CPT staff consisted largely of volunteers, most of them Europeans.

CO: Commanding Officer

Condyles: Distal aspect of long bones such as the femur near the knee, and humerus near the elbow. Both have medial and lateral condyles. The mandible or lower jaw has right and left condyles which articulate with the maxilla or upper jaw. Small bones in the hand and foot also have condyles.

CONUS: Continental United States, used to refer to the homeland, as in, "I'm flying back to CONUS tomorrow."

Cortex: The hard outer aspect of a hollow bone which surrounds the medullary or marrow cavity.

CPT: Clinique Phuoc Thieu, see above.

C-rations: Canned food eaten by soldiers in combat areas. Considered bad-tasting food by most GIs, c-rations or c-rats were a frequent butt of military jokes.

Delayed primary suturing: DPS. This is explained in Chapter three when discussing Field Service Medical School.

Di di mau: Vietnamese for "leaving." Term adopted by US military personnel as in "Let's di di mau" meaning "Let's get out of here."

Dien Bien Phu: Located in Northwest Vietnam, Dien Bien Phu was the site of France's last stand in its unsuccessful "First Indochina War" of 1946–1954. On May 7, 1954, the French garrison of over eleven thousand men was overrun by vastly superior Viet Minh communist forces led by General Vo Nguyen Giap. France's crushing and humiliating defeat at Dien Bien Phu effectively ended the war, with all French forces leaving Southeast Asia shortly thereafter.

Distal: Part of a bone or limb that is far from the trunk, as opposed to "proximal," which is the part closer to the trunk. For example, the proximal aspect of the femur is near the hip, while the distal aspect is near the knee.

DI: Drill instructor. Usually a sergeant, the drill instructor is responsible for training recruits in boot camp. The DI has a reputation for being harsh, relentless, and punitive.

Dust off: also spelled dustoff or dust-off. A term coined in Vietnam circa 1963, it refers to helicopter evacuation of casualties directly from the battlefield.

Dyspnea: An accepted medical term of Greek origin meaning difficult or labored breathing.

ENT: Ear, nose, and throat. A surgical specialty also called Otorhino-laryngology.

ER: Abbreviation for emergency room.

Fellowship: A period of specialized training following formal residency training, fellowship can last one to three years. In orthopedics, for example, a "hand fellowship" will qualify a doctor to perform complex types of hand surgery not covered in regular orthopedic residency training.

Femur: The thighbone, which goes from hip joint to knee joint. Largest long bone in the body.

Femoral: Pertaining to the femur.

Femoral artery: Principal artery supplying the entire lower extremity from groin to toes.

Field Service Medical School (FSMS): A specialized school in boot camp during the Vietnam era, where physicians received instruction in combat surgery and wartime medicine.

First Med: First Medical Battalion, on the outskirts of Danang, was a US Navy-run medical facility equipped with helicopter landing zone, six operating rooms, recovery room, multiple hospital beds as well as a mortuary facility known as "Graves Unit." First Med was dedicated to the treatment of injured or sick United States Marines, and was fully staffed by doctors and corpsmen (who acted as male nurses or orderlies).

Flail chest: When a chest injury causes multiple rib fractures on the same side so that the chest wall collapses. Often lifethreatening, as it can severely impair respiration.

Flipping a graft: When using a vein graft for vascular bypass surgery, the surgeon must "flip" the graft 180 degrees because of the valves inside the vein. The valves are designed to keep blood from backing up in the vein, therefore the graft must be flipped to allow arterial blood to flow freely in the repaired vessel without interference from the valves. Also known as "reversing" a graft.

Fracture reduction: Setting a fracture so that the fracture fragments are in satisfactory position. Fracture reduction is usually followed by application of a cast.

Frag: Short for fragmentation grenade, which on detonation propels hundreds of high velocity fragments in all directions, causing lethal damage. Frag can also be used as a verb, as in, "I'll frag your hootch!"

Fragging: The act of throwing or rolling a fragmentation grenade.

Fragmentation Grenade: See frag.

FSMS: See Field Service Medical School

GI: Short for "Government Issue," GI is used to refer to soldiers in general, and infantrymen in particular.

Giap: General Vo Nguyen Giap, born in 1911, was mandated by Ho Chi Minh to command all communist North Vietnamese forces soon after WWII. He was the military tactical genius who defeated the French at Dien Bien Phu in 1954, then fought the US to a standstill which culminated in the American withdrawal in 1973. Giap then went on to thoroughly defeat the South Vietnamese forces in 1975, with North Vietnam taking over the entire country.

Gook: Defined in Webster's dictionary as "Filipino, Japanese, Korean, etc., gook is a vulgar, offensive term of hostility and contempt. Military slang." Commonly used in Vietnam to refer to any person of Asian descent.

Grunt: Nickname given to the Marine Corps infantryman, possibly because of the sound he makes lifting his heavy pack.

Gunny: Military slang abbreviation for gunnery sergeant.

Hip disarticulation: An amputation through the hip joint, the highest possible level for a lower extremity amputation.

HJD: Hospital for Joint Diseases. A renowned teaching hospital in New York City dedicated to orthopedic surgery and related fields such as rehabilitation medicine, rheumatology, and physical therapy. HJD is famous for its orthopedic residency-training program, where some of the nation's prominent orthopedic surgeons have received their education. HJD and HSS (Hospital for Special Surgery) are considered the two premier orthopedic teaching hospitals in New York City.

Hootch: See author's note in begining of book.

Hotsee bath: A popular Japanese bath where the tub is vertical and one sits on a shelf in hot water up to the neck.

Humerus: Arm bone which goes from shoulder to elbow.

Huss: Military slang for a perk, a break, a benefit or a favor. "When I left Vietnam I got a six day huss," means being allowed to return home from Vietnam after serving only 359 days, or six days short of the mandatory full year.

I-Corps: The US military divided South Vietnam into three major tactical areas marked with Roman numerals: I-Corps, II-Corps, III-Corps. I-Corps, pronounced "eye-corps" to the north, with headquarters in Danang, was where I served. II-Corps was in the middle, and III-Corps to the south.

Incoming: A military term usually yelled out as a warning of impending enemy fire, enemy attack, or enemy rockets. "Incoming!!!" usually meant all personnel should hit the deck or head for cover. Also used as "Incoming brass!" meaning some high-ranking officer was approaching.

In-country: Military term referring to how long one has been in Vietnam. Example: "How long have you been in-country?"

Indochine: or Indochina, French term for Vietnam. "La Guerre d'Indochine" or "the First Indochina War" was fought by France against the communist Viet Minh government headed by Ho Chi Minh, from 1946 through 1954. The war ended with the defeat of the French forces at Dien Bien Phu on May 7, 1954, prior to which Indochina had been a French colony for nearly a hundred years.

Inguinal: Refers to the groin area, as in "inguinal hernia."

Intubation: Placing a breathing tube into someone's trachea to facilitate respiration during anesthesia, or an emergency situation.

IV: Intravenous, placing a needle in a person's vein to maintain hydration, or administer various medications.

IV pole: Pole from which to hang a bottle for IV fluid administration.

KIA: Killed in action or war casualty.

Kuntscher nail: A type of straight, hollow, stainless steel rod used from the 1950s to the 1980s for fixation of femoral shaft fractures. Cloverleaf-shaped in cross section, the Kuntscher nail had great strength and when properly used, it achieved fracture healing in most cases.

Landing zone: A metal plate-covered area for helicopter landing, usually square and about 150×150 feet in size. Also called LZ or landing pad.

Lateral: The outer aspect of a limb or body part, as opposed to medial, which is the inner aspect. The big toe is on the medial side of the foot while the fifth toe is on the lateral side.

Lateral decubitus: A surgical position where the patient is lying on the side with the limb needing surgery facing up.

LCDR: Accepted military abbreviation for lieutenant commander.

Lifer: Slang for a career military person, whether enlisted man or officer. The term lifer is used in contrast to "reservists," who are military personnel drafted for finite, obligatory periods of active military duty.

Lingual: Pertaining to the tongue.

LTJG: Lieutenant Junior Grade, equivalent to Army First Lieutenant.

Long bone: Bones of the arm, leg, hands, and feet, also called tubular bones. As opposed to flat bones such as the skull, ribs, and pelvis.

Lowman clamp: A bone-holding clamp which allows the surgeon to hold and compress fracture fragments together in preparation for metallic fixation.

Lt: Short for Lieutenant.

Mamasan: A perversion of the Japanese, where adding "san" after a name is a show of respect. Mamasan was a name given to any Vietnamese female older than about thirty.

Mandible: Lower jaw.

Mandibular: Pertaining to the mandible.

Maxilla: Upper jaw.

MC: Medical Corps. These initials usually follow the name of an officer to indicate he is a doctor, as in LCDR L.P. Brief (MC), USNR.

Medial: The inner side of a bone or limb, the side toward the body midline. For example, the medial side of the knee is adjacent to the other knee, while the lateral side faces outward.

Mid-rats: Midnight rations, consisting of various snacks provided to hungry troops for consumption late at night.

Military rank: See "officer ranking."

Military time: There is no A.M. or P.M. in military time, which is predicated on a four-digit system of twenty-four hours. 2400 stands for midnight. After midnight the system begins with 0001, which stands for one minute after midnight. 0100 stands for 1 A.M., 0500 is 5 A.M. and 1200 is noon. 1300 is 1 P.M., 1400 is 2 P.M., and so on, all the way up to 2400 midnight, after which the system reverts back to 0000.

Monsoon: Seasonal phenomenon occurring in Southeast Asia characterized by unrelenting, extremely heavy rains and gale force winds.

M16: An assault rifle which became the standard weapon of the American infantry in Vietnam. Firing a 5.54 caliber high-velocity round, light in weight at 5.5 pounds and highly accurate, the M16 has the capacity of firing in single shot mode, as well as semi and fully automatic mode. The M16 has been widely adopted by most Western armed forces.

M60: A heavy machine gun introduced in Vietnam, the M60 fires a 7.62 caliber round arranged on heavy bandoliers which are fed from the left. The empty shells are then ejected from the right side. The M60 essentially replaced the BAR, which was the standard heavy machine gun used by American forces in WWII and Korea.

Nam: Military slang for Vietnam. Also referred-to as "the Nam."

NCO: Non-commissioned officer such as a Sergeant in the Army, or a Chief Petty Officer in the Navy.

Night soil: A farming practice in Asia which utilizes human excrement as fertilizer.

NVA: North Vietnamese Army. Comprised of North Vietnamese regulars, the NVA was also in command of all Vietcong guerillas, and represented the principal fighting force headed by General Giap, the military commander of all communist forces. General Giap answered only to Ho Chi Minh.

Officer ranking: To the civilian population, officer ranking in the US Navy in comparison with the other military branches can be confusing. The following is a listing of equivalent officer ranks with Navy on the left, other branches on the right:

Ensign	Second Lieutenant
Lieutenant Junior Grade	First Lieutenant
Lieutenant	Captain
Lieutenant Commander	Major
Commander	Lieutenant Colonel
Captain	Colonel
Admiral	General

Open fracture: A fracture where the skin is broken. The old term "compound fracture" also meant open fracture but is no longer in use.

OOB: Out of bed.

OR: Common abbreviation for operating room.

OR nurse: Registered nurse trained to function in the operating room in the same capacity as an OR tech. The OR nurse goes through regular nursing school training prior to becoming a specialized OR worker.

OR tech: Operating room technician trained to set up all OR instruments and materials required for surgery. The OR tech also assists the doctor during surgery, then cleans up all instruments and sets up the OR for the following case. The OR tech is usually not a registered nurse.

ORIF: Open reduction and internal fixation. The technique where the orthopedic surgeon makes an incision to expose a fractured bone, puts the fracture fragments together then fixes them with hardware such as screws, plates, wires, pins, nails, rods, or other metallic devices.

Orthopedic surgery: Surgical specialty which treats diseases and injuries of the musculoskeletal system largely excluding the face and skull.

Orthopedist: Orthopedic surgeon. Training includes four years of medical school, then five years of orthopedic surgery residency training. Following that, most orthopedic surgery graduates opt to take one additional year of training known as "fellowship." During fellowship, doctors receive specialized training in one specific orthopedic sub-specialty such as hand or spine.

Orthopod: Another word for orthopedic surgeon.

Osteotome: A type of chisel that tapers to a sharp edge. Osteotomes can vary in width from a quarter inch to two inches, and are used in orthopedic surgery to cut into bone.

Pedal pulse: There are two pedal pulses or foot pulses, which can be palpated on examination. One is the dorsalis pedis pulse on top of the foot, while the other is the posterior tibial pulse found on the inner part of the ankle just below the prominent bony structure called medial malleolus.

Pharynx: Back of the throat.

Pogrom: In late nineteenth and early twentieth century Russia, pogroms were a type of riot where mobs of angry Russians would attack Jews with beatings, rapes, and murders. They would sometimes destroy or set fire to Jewish homes, businesses, and places of worship. Incited by anti-semitism, these pogroms had the overall effect of causing massive Jewish exodus migrations from Russia, mainly to America.

Point man: The first man walking in a single file patrol. Also: "walking point."

Popliteal fossa: Anatomic area in the back of the knee. Important anatomic structures are located there, including the popliteal artery (continuation of the femoral artery), popliteal vein and tibial nerve, as well as important muscles and tendons.

Posterior: The back of a bone or a limb, as opposed to anterior which is the front of a bone or limb.

Postop: After surgery, as in, "the sutures should be removed two weeks postop."

Proximal: Area of a bone or limb located closer to the trunk, as opposed to the distal area located further from the trunk. Example: The proximal area of the arm is located near the shoulder, while the distal area of the arm is closer to the elbow.

PX: A shopping center located on a military base reserved for military personnel. The civilian population usually does not have access to the PX except for dependents and civilian employees of the military base.

Reduce: To set a fracture or dislocation back into place.

Reduction: Setting a fracture. Reduction can either be closed and followed by cast application, or it can be open. In open reduction, the surgeon makes an incision, reduces the fracture fragments to a satisfactory position, then fixes the fragments with some type of metallic hardware.

Relocation: Sometimes used interchangeably with "reduction" for putting a dislocated joint back into place, as in "relocation of a dislocated shoulder." The term reduction is more commonly used.

Respirator: A machine which automatically breathes for patients who are unable to breathe on their own. Also known as a ventilator.

Reveille: From the French, meaning "to wake up," reveille is the name given to the loud melody played in the early morning to wake up troops. Reveille is sounded either by a soldier playing a bugle, or it can be a recording coming out of loudspeaker.

Reversing a graft: Reversing a saphenous vein graft, synonymous with flipping it. See "flipping a graft."

Richardson retractor: A metallic retractor of various sizes used to spread apart or retract soft tissue in order to facilitate the surgeon's view of the operative area.

Round-eye: Military slang for a Caucasian woman pointing out the anatomical difference between Caucasian and Asian eyes.

RPG: Rifle propelled grenade. A grenade shot out of a special rifle, obviating the need to launch the grenade by hand. The short and stocky specialized rifle which fires the grenade can also be referred to as an RPG.

Saphenous vein: The longest vein in the body, the saphenous vein runs on the inner aspect of the leg going from ankle to groin. Located just under the skin, the saphenous vein is often used by vascular surgeons as a graft to replace damaged or diseased arteries.

Sappers: Attackers who use explosive charges rather than firearms to confuse and overcome their intended targets.

Shadchan: Yiddish for matchmaker.

Scrub: The verb "to scrub" means to be working in surgery. The term comes from the act of brushing one's hands clean before going into surgery.

Scrubs: A suit of clothing made up of a short sleeved v-neck pullover shirt and matching pants string-tied at the waist. Worn in the OR by all surgical personnel, scrubs are usually of one standard color for an entire hospital. Scrubs are also often worn by other hospital personnel, especially in the ER.

Scrub tech: Scrubbing technician. The scrub tech is trained to serve in the same capacity as an OR nurse. Same as OR tech.

Seabees: From the initials C.B., which stand for "construction battalion." Seabees are responsible for all construction and structural repair work required at any naval installation.

Shaft fracture: A fracture located anywhere between the uppermost and the lowermost aspects of a long bone. For example, a mid-shaft fracture of the femur is located at or near the middle of the bone.

Shrapnel: A piece of metal varying in size, embedded in an injured soldier's body. Shrapnel usually comes from an exploded bomb, rocket, grenade, or land mine. x-rays are instrumental in helping locate the exact position of shrapnel fragments.

Supracondylar: Above the condyles. In the arm a supracondylar fracture of the humerus occurs just above the elbow joint. In the thigh, a supracondylar fracture of the femur occurs just above the knee joint.

Squawkbox: A type of loudspeaker installed in a hootch for the purpose of rapidly notifying doctors of all emergency situations, mainly incoming casualties.

STAT: From the Latin "statim" meaning "immediately" or "without delay."

Tee tee or Ti ti: From the French "*petit*". A colloquial Vietnamese slang word meaning small, a little, few, not much, scant.

Temporomandibular joint: TMJ. The joint that articulates the lower jaw with the upper jaw, on either side of the face.

THR: Short for total hip replacement.

Thyroid cartilage: The cartilage structure which makes up the Adam's Apple, more prominent in males.

TMJ: Temporomandibular joint. See above.

Torah: The Torah is the central focus of the Jewish faith, both physically and spiritually. Inscribed on a parchment scroll, the Torah contains the five Books of Moses, collectively known as the Pentateuch.

Total hip replacement: A surgical procedure devised by Sir John Charnley of England in the late 1950s, THR consists of replacing the entire hip joint ball-and-socket construct. Various materials can be used for the replacement, but most commonly the new socket (cup, or acetabular component) is made of metal with an inner liner of polyethylene. The new ball (femoral component or stem) is entirely metallic.

Tracheostomy: Opening the windpipe or trachea with a surgical incision and inserting a tube to allow respiration.

Traction: Pulling on a limb with weights, a form of treatment used in certain fractures, currently outmoded.

Triage: French for "sorting." In situations of mass casualties, triage is the art of rapidly assessing each victim and picking the most seriously injured ones for immediate treatment. The triage officer is called upon to make life and death decisions with speed, precision, and sound clinical judgment. Triage is also a noun used interchangeably with ER, as in "Dr. Brief to triage STAT!"

Unit: A military group or outfit. For example, the SEALS are an elite unit of the US Navy, made up of highly trained warriors who are often assigned military tasks of utmost difficulty and risk.

Unit of blood: A standard unit of blood for transfusion measuring 450 cc or approximately one US pint. The adult human body usually contains five liters of blood or approximately eleven units.

USMC: United States Marine Corps

USN: United States Navy. The initials USN usually follow the name of a career naval officer as in Capt. J.W. Lea (MC), USN.

USNR: Unites States Naval Reserve. These initials usually follow the name of a drafted, non-career naval officer, as in LCDR L.P. Brief (MC), USNR.

Vargas Girl: Alberto Vargas (1896–1982) was a noted Peruvian artist famous for painting images which portrayed beautiful, nude or semi-nude women of idealized proportions. *Playboy* began to use his pin-up art in the '60s as "Vargas Girls," making the artist famous. For many years his pin-up art enjoyed wide popularity among men in both the military and civilian worlds.

Vastus medialis: Of the four muscles comprising the quadriceps (rectus femoris, vastus lateralis, vastus medialis, and vastus intermedius), the vastus medialis is the innermost or most medial muscle.

VC: Vietcong.

Vietcong: South Vietnamese guerilla fighters loyal to the communist North. The Vietcong were used by Ho Chi Minh's communist regime to do much of the Vietnam war's "dirty work" such as digging tunnels, terrorizing villagers, and organizing night raids. The Vietcong were also responsible for laying down booby traps such as Claymore or "Bouncing Betty" mines. In the daytime the VC mostly blended with the civilian population, making them very hard to detect. The VC operated mainly at night.

Vil: Abbreviation for village, used mostly by US infantrymen to describe small, countryside villages inhabited by Vietnamese peasants. Frequently infiltrated by the Vietcong, these villages were often blown up by US forces in an effort to ferret out the VC and to gain ground in the war.

Walking point: The man who walks at the front of a jungle patrol. Also known as the "point man."

Water buffalo: A domesticated bovine animal used in Southeast Asian agriculture as a beast of burden. Water buffalo feces were often used in booby trap mines to add wound contamination to the destructive force of the explosive, causing severe infections.

Yarmulke: A round skullcap worn by religious Jews. Also worn by all male Jews whenever they attend religious services in a synagogue or elsewhere.

Yiddish: A dialectic language based principally on German, Yiddish was spoken for centuries by Jewish communities in Central and Eastern Europe until they were decimated by the Holocaust. Yiddish is still spoken by a dwindling number of Holocaust survivors and some of their descendants, as well as by the ultra-orthodox Hasidic population in the US and elsewhere.

Acknowledgements

I owe a debt of gratitude to a number of individuals for their help, encouragement, and inspiration in this work. Although most of what I wrote came directly from my memories of the war and letters sent home, I also conducted informal phone interviews with some of my First Med colleagues, who reminded me of a number of incidents and amusing details I had forgotten.

I am most thankful to my friends and fellow doctors in Vietnam, my war buddies, whose support, kinship, and joviality unquestionably saved my sanity, if not my life. I will go to my grave with undying affection and gratitude for my extended Vietnam "family" in Hootch 8 and First Medical Battalion.

They are: Roger Crumley, Dave Whitney, Sonny Alafriz, Tom Kilroy, Bob Widmeyer, Paul Rubino, Jim Lockhart, Dick Nottingham, Gary Gregersen, Sterling Trenberth, Bob Cave, Bob Rashti, Jehan Mir, and others. I apologize if memory lapses have caused me to leave out any names I should have listed.

Captain Jim Lea, our Skipper, set a shining example of what a commanding officer should be, through his fairness, concern, integrity, and yes, flexibility when it was appropriate.

Dave Lewis, the hero of First Med and rightful recipient of the Navy Cross, who made us all proud, was kind enough to discuss with me the fateful incident of September 24, 1969 in minute detail. I appreciate his permission to include the story in this book.

My partners in orthopedic practice gave me support, especially Dr. Richard Semble, who sat patiently as I read him random chapters from my manuscript and encouraged me with his enthusiastic reception and constructive criticism.

Paul Adler, my good friend and a true political visionary, was kind enough to share with me his take on the significance of the Vietnam War, a vision which puts a new and surprising spin on that conflict's legacy.

My personal transcriptionist Tina Izquierdo sat with me diligently and tirelessly for months, demonstrating remarkable punctuality, integrity, and computer skills. Her tips, good advice, and hard work were instrumental in bringing this project to a successful completion, and are greatly appreciated.

Barry Fixler, my friend and jeweler, is the proudest Marine I have ever known. Kind enough to give me a copy of his own excellent book on Vietnam titled *Semper Cool*, he helped inspire me to write down my own story.

Enrique Ergas, my best friend, confidant, orthopedic colleague par excellence, and comrade in a different war, is a man on whom I can always rely to listen patiently to my problems and give me his best advice.

My wonderful friend Ben Mizrachy not only demonstrated true friendship and kindness upon my return from the war, but through his concern and gentle tenacity, also became a catalyst in the greatest blessing of my life, that of meeting my wife Rochelle.

My mother-in-law Regina Frankel also inspired me to write, as she penned her own memoir describing her suffering in Auschwitz.

My brother Ben and sister Renee lived the ordeal with me. Through their heartwarming letters and news from home, I felt as if they were holding my hand from across the globe.

Sigmund Brief, my father of blessed memory, was a soft-spoken man whose wisdom, wit, and quiet strength I have tried to emulate and teach to my own children.

My mother Itta Brief, of blessed memory, was a woman whose

generosity, unconditional love, perseverance, and courage have inspired and driven me since childhood.

My children Andy, Joanna, James, and Amanda have all heard snippets of my Vietnam stories over the years, especially Amanda at the Vietnam Memorial. They have all exhorted and encouraged me to put my stories in writing, never tiring of hearing details, never complaining of being bored. I am most grateful for their support.

My son-in-law Nick Monsour, for his invaluable skill and assistance in organizing my photo gallery, and for hooking me up with graphic designer Christina Lewis.

Rochelle, my beloved wife of four decades, years ago began encouraging me to overcome my laziness and get down to writing this book. Without her resolve, all the stories and the memories, all the pain and the laughter, all the friends and the nightmares, would have gone unrecorded, doomed to oblivion. But over and above that, Rochelle took an active part in composing, organizing, censoring, editing, and reviewing my text. I could not have gotten through this project without her tireless organizational skills, and for that I am eternally grateful.

My editor Sara Sherbill showed great expertise in streamlining the story, rearranging sequences, and improving my prose to the point of readability.

Finally, thank you to my publisher Matthew Miller, whose remarkable work ethic and thorough professionalism made this book a reality.